KEY NOTES ON
BIOCHEMISTRY AND BIOTECHNOLOGY

For Ready Reference to the

STUDENTS, TEACHERS, RESEARCHERS & ASPIRANTS OF COMPETITIVE EXAMINATIONS

THE EDITORS

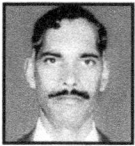

Dr. U.D. Chavan obtained his M.Sc. (Agri. in Biochemistry) degree from Mahatma Phule Krishi Vidyapeeth, Rahuri. He received his Ph.D. degree in Food Science from Memorial University of Newfoundland St. John's Canada in 1999. He has done International Training on "Global Nutrition 2002" at Uppsala University Uppasala, Sweden in 2002. Dr. Chavan worked as Senior Research Assistant in the Department of Biochemistry & Food Science and Technology at MPKV Rahuri from 1988 to 2000. During his Ph.D., he worked as Technician/Research Associate at Atlantic Cool Climate Crop Research Center and Agriculture and Agri-Food Canada. He received D.Sc. degree in 2006 from USA.

Dr. Chavan is presently working as a Senior Cereal Food Technologist in the Department of Food Science & Technology at Mahatma Phule Krishi Vidyapeeth, Rahuri.

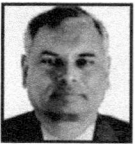

Dr. J.V. Patil obtained his M.Sc. (Agri.) from, MPKV, Rahuri. He completed his course work for Ph.D. at CCSHAU, Hisar and research at MPKV, Rahuri in 1992. He rendered his research and teaching services at MPKV Rahuri as Geneticist, Associate Professor, Plant Breeder and Professor of Genetics & Plant Breeding and Head, Genetics and Plant Breeding Department, MPKV, Rahuri. He also delivered many administrative responsibilities in the University. Dr. Patil joined as the Director, Directorate of Sorghum Research, Hyderabad in August 2010.

THE CONTRIBUTORS

Dr. U.S. Dalvi is an Assistant Professor in the Department of Biochemistry at Mahatma Phule Krishi Vidyapeeth, Rahuri.

Dr. A.S. Jadhav is a Professor of Biotechnology in the Department of Agriculture Botany at Mahatma Phule Krishi Viyapeeth, Rahuri.

KEY NOTES ON
BIOCHEMISTRY AND BIOTECHNOLOGY

For Ready Reference to the

STUDENTS, TEACHERS, RESEARCHERS & ASPIRANTS OF COMPETITIVE EXAMINATIONS

Editors

U.D. CHAVAN

&

J.V. PATIL

Contributors

U.S. DALVI

A.S. JADHAV

2015

Daya Publishing House®

A Division of

Astral International (P) Ltd

New Delhi 110 002

© 2015 PUBLISHER
ISBN: 9789351307020 (International Edition)

Published by	:	**Daya Publishing House®**
		A Division of
		Astral International Pvt. Ltd.
		– ISO 9001:2008 Certified Company –
		4760-61/23, Ansari Road, Darya Ganj
		New Delhi-110 002
		Ph. 011-43549197, 23278134
		E-mail: info@astralint.com
		Website: www.astralint.com
Laser Typesetting	:	**Twinkle Graphics, Delhi**
Printed at	:	**Thomson Press India Limited**

PRINTED IN INDIA

PREFACE

India is an agricultural country. The Indian economy is basically agarian. Inspite of economic and industrialization, agriculture is the backbone of the Indian economy. As Mahatma Gandhi said "India's lives in villages and agriculture is the soul of Indian economy". Agriculture is a vast subject and encompasses at least 20 major and minor subjects in it. New developments have lead to entirely a new face of agriculture. Study of agriculture has always been intrigued with a mosaic of interwove concepts, subjects, facts and figures. There are number of books and large literature on Biochemistry and Biotechnology but the Key Notes type of book have not been compiled in a readable manner.

The present book *"Key Notes on Biochemistry and Biotechnology"* has been designed to fulfill this long felt need of students, teachers, researchers and aspirants of competitive examinations. It is designed in such a way that give rapid, easy access to the core materials in a short format which facilitates easily learning and rapid revision. The book carries fundamentals of The book is divided into two part. Part A is Biochemistry and Part B of the Book is on Biotechnology. The most recent information is provided along with a detailed list of references for further reading.

Hope this book would be highly useful for graduate and post-graduate students of agriculture, teachers and researchers. This book will also useful for the aspirants of various competitive examinations such as Agricultural Research Service (ARS), ICAR- National Eligibility Test (NET), State Eligibility Test (SET), Junior Research Fellowship (JRF), Senior Research Fellowship (SRF), Civil Services, Allied Agricultural Examinations and Extension Workers for reference and easy answers of many complicated questions. Thus it is expected that this book will adequately meet the need of wider circle of students and readers for preparing their professional career.

We acknowledge the references that are used in this manuscript. Authors are also thankful to all scientists and friends who have helped directly or indirectly while preparing this manuscript. The editors of grateful to all the contributors for their cooperation, support and timely submission of their manuscripts for bringing out this publication. We would have like to acknowledge the patience and support of our families whilst we have spent many hours with drafts of manuscripts rather than with them. Lastly, our sincere thanks to publisher Astral International Pvt. Ltd., New Delhi who provides an opportunity to publish this book.

To all readers we extend an invitation to report that no doubts have escaped our attention and to offer suggestion for improvements that can be incorporated in future editions.

U.D.Chavan and J.V. Patil

Editors

CONTENTS

PART–A

BIOCHEMISTRY

1

DISCOVERIES

Year	Scientist	Discovery
1665	Robert Hook	The term cell was used
1674	Leewenhook	Discovered free cell
1743	Lavoisier	Father of modern chemistry
1770	Pristley	Discovery of O_2 as a byproduct of plant respiration
1773	Routle	Isolated Urea from Urine
1780	Esvoisier	O_2 is involved in animal respiration
1783	Spallanzani	Digestion of protein is a chemical process
1783	Spallanzani	Digestion of protein is a chemical process
1813	Claude Bemard	Physical chemistry
1822	Louis Pasture	Molecular structure of organic compound
1828	Wholler	Synthesis of urea from inorganic material
1830	Warburg, Wieland, Keilin and Theorell	Enzymes, cofactors involved in cellular oxidation
1830	Kerbs	TCA Cycle (Tricarboxylic Acid)
1830	Liebig	Heat generated in the body as a result of combustion of food, the man eat.
1838	Schleiden	Cell theory. Cell is fundamental unit.
1842	Mayer	First law of thermodynamics is also obeyed by living cells
1855	Virchow	Omnis cellulase
1859	Van't Hoff & Arrehmius	Interpretation of living organisms
1866	Mendel	Law of inheritance
1869	Darwin	Evolution of life
1871	Meischer	Isolated nuclei from structure known as DNA from WBC
1875	Hertwig	Sperm cell nuclei and egg cell nuclei fusion are occurred during fertilization
1880	Felming	Cell ensures continuity in one generation to other by mechanism of mitosis
1890	Waldeyer	Precise chromosome partitioning
1900	Emil-Fischer	Systematic study of enzymes
1901	Correns, Tschermeck and Devries	Independently discovered Mendel's law
1903	Neuberg	Word as Biochemistry given by him
1926	Summer	Isolated enzyme urease from Jackbean seed

contd...

Year	Scientist	Discovery
1930	Northron	Isolation of digestive enzymes; pepsin and Trypsin.
1940	Beadle and Tatum	One gene one enzyme hypothesis
1944	Avery and Leoad	DNA is genetic material
1950	Pauling	Structure of fibrous proteins.
1950	Erwin Chargaff	Found that the ratios of adenine to thymine and guanine to cytosine in DNA were nearly 1.0 in all species studied.
1953	Nirenburg and Ochoa	Discovered genetic code
1953	Korn berg	Enzymatic synthesis of DNA
1953	Sanger	First complete amino acid sequence of protein.
1955	Wetson and Crick	Structure of DNA
1961	Jacob and Monod	Gene regulation
1979	Igenhousz	Importance of light in Photosynthesis

2

ABBREVIATIONS

Short Form	Full Form
Ab	Antibody
DE'_o	Change in redoxpotential under standard conditions
G	Gibbs Free Energy
DG^{++}	Gibbs Energy of Activation
$DG^{o'}$	Gibbs free energy under standard conditions
2, 4-D	2, 4-Dichlorophenoxyacetic acid
2-ip	Isopentenyl adenine
5-BUdR	5-Bromodeoxyuridine
ABA	Abscisic acid
ACAT	Acy-CoA Cholesterol Acyl Transferase
ACC	1-Aminocyclopropane-1-carboxylic acid
ACMV	African cassava mosaic virus
ACP	Acyl Carrier Protein
ADA	Adenosine deaminase
ADP	Adenosine Diphosphate
Ag	Antigen
AG-LCR	Asymmetric gap ligase chain reaction
AGP	Araribinogalactan protein
AIDS	Acquired Immuno Deficiency Syndrome
ALA	Amino Laevulinic Acid
Ala	Alanine
AMP	Adenosine monophosphate
ANF	Atrial natriuretic factor
Arg	Arginine

Short Form	Full Form
ARS	Autonomously replicating sequences
Asn	Asparagine
Asp	Aspartate
ATCase	Aspartate trans carbamoylase
ATCC	American Type Culture Collection
ATL	Adult T-cell Leukemia
ATP	Adenosine 5'-triphosphate
ATPase	Adenosine triphosphate
AZT	Azidothymidine
BCG	Bacillus of Calmette Guerien
BHC	Benzene hexachloride
BMV	Brome mosaic virus
BOD	Biochemical oxygen demand
bp	Base pairs
BPV	Bovine papilloma virus
BSC	Bundle sheath Cells
cAMP	3'.5' cyclic AMP
CaMV	Cauliflower mosaic virus
CAP	Catabolite Activator Protein
CCMV	Chrysanthmum chlorotic mottle virus
cDNA	Complementary Deoxyribonucleic acid
CDP	Cytidine Diphosphate
CDR	Complement determining region
CEA	Carcinoembryonic antigen
CEN	Centromere
CFSTR	Continuous flow stirred tank reactor
cGMP	Cyclic Guanosine monophosphate
CGT	Cyclodextrin glucosyltransferase
CH	Constant region of heavy chain (antibodies)
CHEFE	Countour clamped homogeneous electric field electrophoresis

Short Form	Full Form
CHS	Chalcone synthase
CL	Constant region of light chain (antibodies)
cM	CentiMorgan
CM	Carboxymethyl
CMP	Cytidine monophosphate
CMS	Cytoplasmic male sterility
CMV	Cucumber mosaic virus
CNBr	Cyanogen Bromide
CoA	Coenzyme A
COD	Chemical oxygen demand
CoQ	Cytochrome Q (ubiquinone)
$CoQH_2$	Ubiquinol
cos	Cohesive sequence
COS	Cv1 origin of SV40 (Cv1 is a monkey cell line)
CP	Coat protein
cpDNA	Chlooroplast DNA
CpG	Cyclopentadienyl guanosine
C-region	Constant region
CSIR	Council for Scientific and Industrial Research
CSL	Corn Steep Liquor
CSV	Chrysanthemum stunt virus
CTL	Cytotoxic T Lymphocyte
CTP	Cytosine Trihosphate
Cys	Cysteine
d	2'-deoxyribo-
DAG	1,2-diacylglycerol
dATP	Deoxyadenosine 5'-triphosphate
dCTP	Deoxycytidine triphosphate
dCTP	Deoxycytidine 5'-triphosphate
ddATP	2', 3'-dideoxyadenosine triphosphate

Short Form	Full Form
ddCTP	2', 3'-deoxycytidine triphosphate
ddGTP	2', 3'-dideoxyguanosine triphosphate
ddNTP	Dideoxynucleoside triphosphate
ddTTP	2', 3'-dideoxythymidine triphosphate
DEAE	Diethylaminoethyl
DFR	Dihydroflavanol 4-reductase
dGTP	Deoxyguanosine triphosphate
dGTP	Deoxyguanosine 5'-triphosphate
DH	Doubled haploid
DHFR	Dihydrofolate reductase
DHK	Dihydrokaempferol
DIMBOA	2,4-Dihydroxy-7-methoxy-1, 4-benzoxazin-3-one
DIPF	Diisopropylfluorophosphate
DME	Dulbecco's enriched modification of minimal essential medium
DMSO	Dimethyl sulphoxide
DNA	Deoxyribonucleic acid
DNase	Doxyribonuclease
DNP	2,4-dinitrophenol
DOPE	Dioleoyl phosphatidylethanolamine
DSP	Downstream processing
DTA	Diphtheria Toxin A Chain
dTTP	Deoxythymidine 5'-triphosphate
E	Redox Potential
EBR	Fluidized bed reactor
EC	Enzyme Commission
EDTA	Ethylene diamine tetra-acetic acid
EF	Elongation Factor
EGF	Epidermal Growth Factor
EIA	Enzyme immuno assay
eIF	Eukaryotic Initation Factor

Short Form	Full Form
ELISA	Enzyme Linked Immunosorbent Assay
EMIT	Enzyme multiple immuno assay technique
EPO	Erythropoietin
EPR	Electron paramagnetic resonance
EPSPS	5-enolpyruvyl-3-phosphoshikimic acid synthase
ER	Endoplasmic Reticulum
ES	Embryonic stem cells
ESPS	5-enolpyruvyl shikimate-3-phosphate synthase
EST	Expression sequence tags
F-2,6-BP	Fructose 2,6-bisphosphate
FAB	Fragment with antigen binding (of antibodies)
FACS	Fluorescence activated cell sorter
FDA	Fluorescein diacetate
FAD	Flavin Adenine Dinucleotide (Oxidized)
$FADH_2$	Flavin Adenine Dinucleotide (Reduced)
FBPase	Fructose Bisphosphatase
Fc	Crystal forming fragment (of antibodies)
FGF	Fibroblast growth factor
FID	Fluorescence immuno assay
FISH	Fluorescence *in situ* hybridization
FLV	Feline leukemia virus
FMD	Foot and mouth disease
FMN	Flavin Mononucleotide (Oxidized)
$FMN\ H_2$	Flavin Mononucleotide (Reduced)
FR	Framework region
FSH	Follicle stimulating hormone
G/cNAc	N-acetyl glucosamine
Ga/NAc	N-acetyl galactosamine
GA_3	Gibberellic acid
GDP	Guanosine diphosphate

Short Form	Full Form
GEM	Genetically engineered micro-organism
G-LCR	Gap-ligase chain reaction
Gln	Glutamine
Glu	Glutamate
Gly	Glycine
GMP	Guanosine Mono Phosphate
GOGAT	Glutamate synthase
GOX	Glyphasate oxidoreductase
GPI	Glycosyl phophatidyl Inositol
GR	Growth regulator
GTP	Guanosine 5'-triphosphate
HART	Hybrid arrested translation
HAT medium	Hypoxanthine aminopterin and thymidine medium
Hb	Hemoglobin
Hbs	Sickle Cell Hemoglobin
HBsAg	Hepatitis B surface antigen
hCG	Human chorionic gonadotropin
HDL	High Density Lipoprotein
HEPA filter	High efficiency particulate air filter
HGF	Hepatocyte growth factor
HGH	Human growth hormone
HGPRT	Hypoxanthine-guanine phosphoribosyl transferase
His	Histidine
HIV	Human Immunodeficiency Virus
hMG	Human menopausal gonadotropin
HMG	3-hydroxy-3-methyl glutaryl
HMM	Heavy meromyosin
hr	Hours
HSP	Heat Shock Protein
HSV	Herpes simplex virus

Short Form	*Full Form*
HSV-tk	Herpes simplex virus thymidine kinase
HTLV-1	Human T-cell leukemia lymphoma virus-1
Hyl	5-hydroxylysine
IAA	Indole-3-acetic acid
IAM	Indole-3-acetamide
IARI	Indian Agricultural Research Institute
IBA	Indole-3-butyric acid
ICAR	Indian Council of Agricultural Research, New Delhi
ICGEB	International Centre for Genetic Engineering and Biotechnology
IDL	Intermediate Density Lipoprotein
IF	Initiation Factor
Ig	Immunoglobulin
IGF	Insulin like growth factor
IgG	Immunoglobin G
IL	Interleukin
IL-2	Interleukin-2
Ile	Isoleucine
IMDM	Iscoves modified Dulbecco's medium
INF	Interferon
IP_3	Inositol 1,4,5-triphosphate
IPTG	Isopropyl-Beta-D-thiogalactopyranoside
IS	Insertion sequence
ISH	*In situ* hybridization
IV	Intermediate vector
IVRI	Indian Veterinary Research Institute
K	Equilibrium Constant
kb	Kilo base pairs
kg	Kilogram
K_m	Michaelis Constant
l	Litre

Short Form	Full Form
LAK Cells	Lymphokine activated killer cells
LCAT	Lecithin-Cholesterol-Acyltransferase
LCR	Ligase chain reaction
LDH	Lactate Dehydrogenase
LDL	Low Density Lipoprotein
Leu	Leucine
LGL	Large granular lymphocyte
LH	Luteinising hormone
LMM	Light Meromyosin
LN	Liquid nitrogen
LRE	Light response element
Lys	Lysine
M	Molar (= gram molecular weight)
m mol 1^{-1}	Milli mole per litre
Mab	Monoclonal antibody
Mb	Mega base pairs (10^6 bp)
MC	Mesophyll cells
MEM	Minimal essential medium
Met	Methionine
min	Minutes
MLV	Moloney murine leukemia virus
mM	Milli molar (= mg molecular weight)
mol	Gram molecular weight
mRNA	Messenger Ribonucleic Acid
MSV	Maize streak virus
mtDNA	Mitochondrial DNA
Mtx	Methotrexate
NAA	Naphthalene acetic acid
NAD	Nicotinamide adenine dinucleotide
NAD$^+$	Nicotinamide Adenine Dinucleotide (Oxidized)

Short Form	Full Form
NADH	Nicotinamide adenine dinucleotide (reduced)
NADP⁺	Nicotinamide Adenine Dinucleotide Phosphate (Oxidized)
NADPH	Nicotinamide Adenine Dinucleotide Phospate (Reduced)
NAM	N-acetylmuramic Acid
NBPGR	National Bureau of Plant Genetic Resources
NBTB	National Biotechnology Board
NCL	National Chemical Laboratory
NDRI	National Dairy Research Institute
N-f Met	N-Formyl Methionine
NGF	Nerve growth factor
NHP	Nonhistone Protein
NIL	Near isogenic lines
NIR	Near infrared spectroscopy
NK cells	Natural killer cells
NMR	Nuclear magnetic resonance
OSRV	Odontoglossum-ringspot virus
p.s.i.	Pounds per square inch
PAGE	Polyacrylamide gel electrophoresis
PALA	N-Phosphonacetyl-L-aspartate
PBR	Packed bed reactor
PC	Phosphatidyl choline
PC	Plasto Cyanin
PCB's	Polychlorinated biphenyls
PCR	Polymerase Chain Reaction
PDGF	Platelet-derived growth factor
PEG	Polyethylene glycol
PEP	Phosphoenol Pyruvate
PFGE	Pulsed field gel electrophoresis
PFK	Phosphofructo Kinase
Pg	Picogram

Short Form	Full Form
PG	Polygalacturonase
PGA	Phosphoglyceric acid
PHB	Polyhydroxy butyrate
Phe	Phenylalanine
Pi	Inorganic phosphate
PI	Isoelectric Point
PK	Dissociation Constant
PMSG	Pregnant mare serum gonadotropin
ppb	Parts per billion
PPi	Inorganic Pyrophosphate
ppm	Parts per million
PQ	Plastoquinone
Pro	Proline
PS	Pedigree selection
PS-I	Photo System I
PS-II	Photo System II
PTH	Phenylthiohydantoin
PVC	Polyvinyl carbonate
PVP	Polyvinyl pyrrolidon
PVS	Potato virus S
PVX	Potato virus X
PYAC	Yeast artificial yeast chromosome vector
Q	Ubiquinone (Coenzyme Q)
QH_2	Ubiquinol
QTL	Quantitative trait loci
r.p.m.	Revolutions per minute
RAPD	Randomly amplified polymorphic DNAs
RER	Rough Endoplasmic Reticulum
RF	Release Factor/Response Factor
RFLP	Restriction fragment length polymorphism

Short Form	Full Form
RIA	Radio immuno assay
RNA	Ribonucleic Acid
RNAase	Ribonuclease
rRNA	Ribosomal RNA
RSV	Rous sarcoma virus
RTF	Resistance transfer factor
RuBISCO	Ribulose 1,5-bisphosphate carboxylase/oxygenase
rubisco	Ribulose Bisphosphate Carboxylase
s	Seconds
SCID	Severe combined immune deficiency
SCP	Single cell protein
SDS	Sodium Dodecyl Suphate
SE	Somatic embryo
Ser	Serine
SER	Smooth Endoplasmic Reticulum
snoRNA	Small Nucleolar RNA
snoRNP	Small Nuclear Ribonucleo Protein
snRNA	Small Nuclear RNA
SRP	Signal Recognition Particle
SSB	Single Stranded DNA binding (protein)
SSBP	Single strand binding protein
SSD	Single cell protein
SSR	Short sequence repeats
STMS	Sequence tagged micro satellite sites
STR	Stirred tank reactor
STS	Sequence tagged sites
SV 40	Simian virus 40
TAV	Tomato aspermy virus
TBGRI	Tropical Botanical Garden and Research Institute
TBP	TATA box-binding protein

Short Form	Full Form
T-DNA	Transferred DNA
TERI	Tata Energy Research Institute
TFII	Transcription Factor for RNA Polymerase II
TGF-b	Transforming growth factor b
Thr	Threonine
Tk	Thymidine kinase
T_m	Melting point
TMGMV	Tobacco mild green mosaic virus
TMV	Tobacco mosaic virus
TNF	Tumour necrosis factor
TobRV	Tobacco ringspot virus
ToMV	Tobacco mosaic virus
tPA	Tissue plasminogen activator
tRNA	Transfer RNA
Trp	Tryptophan
TTC	2,3,5-Triphenyl tetrazolium chloride
Tyr	Tyrosine
UDP	Uridine diphosphate
UMP	Uridine monophosphate
UNO	United Nations Organization
UTP	Uridine triphosphate
UV	Ultraviolet (light)
V/V	Volume by volume
Val	Valine
VH	Variable region of heavy chain (antibodies)
VL	Variable region of light chain (antibodies)
VLDL	Very Low Density Lipoprotein
V_{max}	Maximum Rate of Reaction
VNTR	Variable number of tandem repeats
V_o	Initial Rate of Reaction

Short Form	Full Form
VP 1,2 or 3	Virion protein 1, 2 or 3
V-region	Variable region (in antibodies)
VS	Volatile solids
VV	Vaccinia virus
W/V	Weight by volume
W/W	Weight by weight
WDA	Wheat dwarf virus
x	Genomic chromosome number
XGPRT	Xanthine-guanine phosphoribosyl transferase
YCP	Yeast centromere plasmids
YEP	Yeast episomal plasmids
YIP	Yeast integrative plasmids
YRP	Yeast replicating plasmids

3

DEFINITIONS

Term	Definition
Abiotic	Pertaining to nonliving environmental factors, such as temperature, light, water and nutrients.
Abscisic acid (ABA)	A plant hormone that generally acts to inhibit growth, promote dormancy, and help the plant withstand stressful conditions.
Absorption spectrum	The range of a pigment's ability to absorb various wavelengths of light.
Acid	According to the Bronsted definition, any ion or molecule, which can furnish a proton to solution.
Acclimation	Physical adjustment to a change in an environmental factor.
Acetyl CoA	The entry compound for the Krebs cycle in cellular respiration, formed from a fragment of pyruvate attached to a coenzyme.
Activation energy	The energy, Ea, defined by the Arrhenius equation. $R = Ae^{-Et}/RT$, Which is interpreted as the difference between the average energy of the reactant molecules and the energy required to form the reactive intermediate (activated complex) which leads to product.
Active site	A region on the surface of an enzyme which specifically binds the substrate and which facilitates the reaction of the substrate to form product.
Activity	The "thermodynamically effective" concentration of a substrate. Its value depends upon the choice of a standard state for the substrate referred to. For solutes, the standard state is often taken as 1 M concentration, and the activity of the solute is approximately equal to the molar concentration in vary dilute solutions. For solvents the standards state is taken as the pure solvent, and the activity of a solvent in dilute solution is approximately unity.

Term	Definition
Activation energy	The energy Ea, defined by the Arrhenius equation. $R = A_e^{-Ea}/RT$, which is interpreted as the difference between the average energy of the reactant molecules and the energy required to form the reactive intermediate (activated complex) which leads to product.
Acquired character	A change from the normal type brought about by environmental influence.
Acquired immunity	The type of immunity achieved when antigens enter the body the body naturally or artificially. Acquired immunity is due to stimulation of antibody production and production of memory cells keyed to the antigen.
Actin	A globular protein that links into chains, two of which twist helically about each other, forming microfilaments in muscle and other contractile elements in cells.
Activator	Some enzymes have binding sites for small molecules that stimulate their activity; these stimulator molecules are called activators.
Active transport	Active transport of a molecule across a membrane against its concentration gradient requires an input of metabolic energy. In the case of ATP-derive active transport, the energy required for the transport of the molecule (Na^+, K^+, Ca^{++}, or H^+) across the membrane is derived from the coupled hydrolysis of ATP (e.g., Na^+/K^+- ATPase). If both the molecule to be transported and the ion move in the same direction across the membrane, the process is called symport (e.g., Na^+/glucose transporter). If the molecule and the ion move in opposite directions it is called antiport (e.g., erythrocyte band 3 anion transporter).
Activity	The "thermodynamically effective" concentration of a substrate.
Active site	A region on the surface of an enzyme which specifically binds the substrate and which facilitates the reaction of the substrate to form product.
Adaptation	Modification of an organism fitting it more perfectly to conditions of its environment.
Adenine/Guanine	Nitrogen base one of two purines found in both DNA and RNA.

Term	Definition
Adenosine triphosphate (ATP)	The main energy currency for cells. ATP energy is used to promote ion pumping enzyme activity and muscular contraction.
Adipsin	A protein that appears to be made adipose cells and acts as a communication link between adipose cells and the brain.
Aerobic respiration	Harvesting chemical energy in the form of ATP from food molecules, with oxygen as the final electron acceptor.
AIDS	The name of the late stage of HIV infection; deficiency by a specific reduction of T cells and the appearance of characteristic secondary infections.
Aldehyde	An organic molecule with a carbonyl group located at the end of the carbon skeleton.
Aleurone	Protein matter in the form of grains occurring in the endosperm of ripe seeds.
Allele	One of two normally alternate forms of a gene one being the normal wild type (+), the other the mutant type.
Allopolyploid	A common type of polyploid species resulting from two different species interbreeding and combining their chromosomes.
Alpha (α) helix	A spiral shape constituting one form of the secondary structure of proteins, arising from a specific hydrogen-bonding structure.
Amino acid	The building block for proteins containing a central carbon atom with a nitrogen atom and other atoms attached OR an organic molecule possessing both carboxyl and amino groups. Amino acids serve as the monomers of proteins.
Amino acid codons	Val = GUA, Phe = UUU, Lys = AAA, Gly = GGA, Ser = UCC, Arg = AGA, Pro = CCC, Glu = GAA, Leu = UUG, Ala = GCA, Trp = UGG, Met = AUG.
Anabolic pathway	A metabolic pathway that consumes energy to build complicated molecules from simpler ones.
Anabolic reactions	The reactions by which the structural and functional components of the cell are synthesized.

Term	Definition
Anaerobic respiration	A form of respiration that occurs in a few groups of bacteria living in anaerobic environments such as soil, the final electron acceptors are sulphate and nitrate.
Analogy	The similarity of structure between two species that are not closely related; attributable to convergent evolution.
Anaphase	A stage in cell division following metaphase in which the daughter chromosomes, pass from the equatorial plate in metaphase midway to the two poles at the opposite ends of the cell.
Angstrom (Å)	A unit of length equal to 10^{-8} cm.
Anhydride	A compound formed by the loss of water between two acids
Anion	A negatively charged ion.
Anther	In seed plants the part of the stamen where pollen grains (microspores) are formed.
Anthocyanin	A soluble glucoside pigment producing either reddish or purplish colour to flowers and other parts of plants.
Antibiotic	A chemical that kills or inhibits the growth of bacteria, often via transcriptional or translational regulation.
Antibody	An antigen-binding immunoglobulin produced by B cells, that functions as the effectors in an immune response; or the capacity of proteins to distinguish among different molecules or immunoglobulins than in enzymes. Antibodies are valuable tools for identifying and purifying proteins.
Anticodon	A specified base triplet on one end of a tRNA molecule that recognizes a particular complementary codon on an mRNA molecule.
Antigen	A substance (usually a protein) capable of stimulating antibody production when introduced into an animal body.
Apoferritin	A protein in the intestinal cell that binds with the ferric form of iron (Fe^{+3}) to form ferritin.
Aqueous solution	A solution in which water is the solvent.
Asymmetric carbon	A carbon atom covalently bonded to four different atoms or groups of atoms.

Term	Definition
Atherosclerosis	Atherosclerosis is characterized by cholesterol rich arterial thickenings (atheromas) that narrow the arteries and cause blood clots to form. If these blood clots block the coronary arteries supplying the heart, the result is a myocardial infarction or heart attack.
Atomic number	The number of protons in the nucleus of an atom, unique for each element and designated by a subscript to the left of the elemental symbol.
Atomic weight	The total atomic mass, which is the mass in grams of one mole of the atom.
Autosomes	Chromosomes other than sex chromosomes.
Autotrophic nutrition	A mode of obtaining organic food molecules without eating other organisms. Autotrophus use energy from the sun or from the oxidation of inorganic substances to make organic molecules from inorganic ones.
Auxins	A class of plant hormones, including indolacetic acid, that has a variety of effects, such as phototropic response through stimulation of cell elongation, stimulation of secondary growth and development of leaf trances and fruit.
Avidin	A protein found in raw egg whites that can bind biotin and inhibit its absorption. Cooking destroys avidin.
B cell	A type of lymphocyte that develops in the bone marrow and later produces antibodies, which mediate humoral immunity.
Barr body	The dense object that lies along the inside of the nuclear envelope in cell of female mammals, representing the one inactivated X chromosome.
Basal body	A cell structure identical to a centriole that organizes and anchors the microtubule assembly of a cilium or flagellum.
Basal metabolic rate (BMR)	The minimum number of kilocalories a resting animal requires to fuel itself for a given time.
Base	According to the Bronsted definition, any ion or molecule, which can accept a proton.
Beta (b) plated sheet	A zigzag shape constituting one form of the secondary structure of proteins formed of hydrogen bonds between polypeptide segments running in opposite directions.

Term	Definition
Bile salts	Bile salts (bile acids) are the major excretory form of cholesterol. These polar compounds are formed in the liver by converting cholesterol into the activated intermediate cholyl CoA and then combining this compound with either glycine to form glycocholate or taurine to form taurocholate. The detergent-like bile salts are secreted into the intestine where they aid the digestion and uptake of dietary lipids.
Bioavailability	The degree to which the amount of an ingested nutrient actually gets absorbed and so is available to the body.
Biochemical genetics	The branch of genetics concerned with the inheritance of genetic differences in the ability or inability to synthesize or metabolize certain chemicals.
Biochemistry	Biochemistry is defined as it deals with chemical processing in living matter from smallest to biggest organisms.
Biological value	The body's ability to retain nutrient absorbed from a food.
Biotechnology	The use of advanced scientific techniques to alter and ideally improve characteristics of animals and plants.
Biotic	Pertaining to the living organisms in the environment such as pests, insects, birds, bacteria fungus etc.
Blood brain barrier	A specialized capillary arrangement in the brain that restricts the passage of most substances into the brain, thereby preventing dramatic fluctuations in the brain's environment.
Blood pressure	The hydrostatic force that blood exerts against the wall of a vessel.
Bond energy	The quantity of energy that must be absorbed to break a particular kind of chemical bond equal to the quantity of energy the bond releases when it forms.
Bottleneck effect	Genetic drift resulting from reduction of a population, typically by a natural disaster, such that the surviving population is no longer genetically representative of the original population.
Bowman's capsule	A cup-shaped receptacle in the vertebrate kidney that is the initial, expanded segment of the nephron where filtrate enters from the blood.

Term	Definition
Buffer	A substance that consists of acid and base forms in solution and that minimizes changes in pH when extraneous acids or bases are added to the solution.
Calorie	The amount of heat energy required raising the temperature of one gram of water from 14.5 to 15.5°C.
Carcinogen	Any cancer-inducing substance.
Catabolic reaction	The reactions by which substrates are degraded to simpler substances in the cell
Catalyst	A substance that change the rate of a chemical reaction, usually accelerating it. The catalyst is not consumed in the process, nor does it affect the equilibrium constant of the reaction.
CDNA clone	A selected host cell with a vector containing a cDNA molecule from another organism.
C_3 plant	A plant that uses the Calvin cycle for the initial steps that incorporate CO_2 in to organic material, forming a three-carbon compound as the first stable intermediate.
C_4 plant	A plant that prefers the Calvin cycle with reactions that incorporate CO_2 into four carbon compounds, the end product of which supplies CO_2 for the Calvin cycle.
Calorie	The amount of heat energy required to raise the temperature of 1 g of water 1°C; the amount of heat energy that 1 g of water releases when it cools by 1°C. The Calorie (with a capital C), usually used to indicate the energy content of food, is a kilocalorie.
Calvin cycle	The second of two major stages in photosynthesis (following the light reactions), involving atmospheric CO_2 fixation and reduction of the fixed carbon into carbohydrate.
CAM plant	A plant that uses crassulacean acid metabolism, an adaptation for photosynthesis in arid conditions, first discovered in the family Crassulaceae. Carbon dioxide entering open stomata during the night is converted into organic acids, which release CO_2 for the Calvin cycle during the day, when stomata are closed.
Capsid	The protein shell that encloses the viral genome; rod-shaped, polyhedral, or more completely shaped.

Term	*Definition*
Carbohydrate	A sugar (monosaccharide) or one of its dimmers (disaccharides) or polymers (polysaccharides).
Carbon fixation	The initial incorporation of carbon dioxide into organic compounds.
Carbonyl group	A functional group present in aldehydes and ketones, consisting of a carbon double bonded to an oxygen atom.
Carboxyl group	A functional group present in organic acids, consisting of a single carbon atom double bonded to an oxygen atom and also bonded to a hydroxyl group.
Carcinogen	A chemical agent that causes cancer.
Carnivore	An animal, such as a shark, hawk or spider that eats other animals.
Carrier protein	A transport protein involved in facilitated diffusion, possessing a specific binding site for a specific substance.
Cartilage	A type of flexible connective tissue with an abundance of collagenous fibers embedded in chondrin.
Catabolic pathway	A metabolic pathway that releases energy by breaking down complex molecules into simpler compounds.
Catabolite activator protein (CAP)	In *E. coli*, a helper protein that stimulates gene expression by binding within the promoter region of an operaon and enhancing the promoter's ability to associate with RNA polymerase.
Cation	An ion with a positive charge, produced by the loss of one or more electrons.
Cation exchange	A process in which positively charged minerals are made available to plant when hydrogen ions in the soil displace mineral ions from the clay particles.
Cell adhesion molecules (CAMs)	A diverse group of molecules on the surface of cells that contribute to selective cell association during embryonic development.
Cell	The basic unit of life. The smallest unit capable of independent reproduction.
Cell wall	Unique to plant cells, a wall formed of cellulose fibers embedded in a polysaccharide protein matrix. The primary cell wall is thin and flexible, whereas the secondary cell wall is stronger and more rigid and the primary constituent of wood.

Term	Definition
Cellular respiration	The most prevalent and efficient catabolic pathway for the production of ATP, in which oxygen is consumed as a reactant along with the organic fuel.
Cellulose	A structural polysaccharide of cell walls, consisting of glucose monomers joined by b–1, 4-glycosidic linkages.
Central nervous system (CNS)	In vertebrate animals, the brain and spinal cord.
Chemiosmosis	The ability of certain membranes to use chemical energy to pump hydrogen ions and then harness the energy stored in the H^+ gradient to drive cellular work, including ATP synthesis.
Chemoautotroph	An organism that needs only carbon dioxide as carbon source but that obtains energy by oxidizing inorganic substances.
Chemoheterotrop	An organism that must consume organic molecules both for energy and carbon.
Chemical equilibrium	The rates of the forward and reverse reactions become equal, so that the concentrations of reactants and products stop changing such type of mixture is said to be chemical equilibrium.
Chitin	A structural polysaccharide of an amino sugar found in many fungi and in the exoskeletons of all arthropods.
Chlorophyll	A green pigment located within the chloroplasts of plants; chlorophyll a can participate directly in the light reactions, which convert solar energy to chemical energy.
Chloroplasts	Chlorophyll-containing structures found in the cytoplasm of green plant cells. Photosynthesis takes place in the chloroplasts.
Cholesterol	A steroid forming an essential component of animal cell membranes and acting as a precursor molecule for the synthesis of other biologically important steroids.
Chromogene	A heredity determiner in the chromosome in contrast to determiners in the cytoplasm.
Chromosome	A filamentous body in the cell nucleus, which is conspicuous during certain stages of cell division. The chromosomes of the cell contain the genes; or A deep staining, rod like body in the nucleus of cells, visible at cell division. Chromosomes contain the genes, the hereditary determiners. All species have characteristic chromosome numbers.

Term	Definition
Clone	A lineage of genetically identical individuals.
Codon	A group of three bases in fact codes for one amino acid. This group of bases is called as codon. UAG, UAA and UGA are the only three codons that do not specify an amino acid. The genetic code is non-overlapping. Codons that specify the same amino acid are called synonyms; e.g., CAU and CAC are synonymous for the histidine. Most synonymous differ only in the last base of the triplet.
Coenzymes	A small molecular weight substance required for the catalytic activity of one or group of enzymes; or an enzyme often contains a tightly bound small molecule, termed a coenzyme that is essential for the activity of the enzyme.
Cofactor	Synonymous with coenzyme. Often used to refer to a substance of unknown structure.
Colour blindness	Inability to distinguish certain colours.
Complete proteins	Proteins that contain ample amounts of all nine/eight essential amino acids.
Competitive inhibitor	An inhibitor of an enzymatic reaction whose inhibition can be abolished by high concentrations of substrate. In other words the maximum velocity is the same in the presence and absence of the inhibitor. This effect is usually interpreted in terms of a competition between the inhibitor and the substrate for the active site of the enzyme.
Complementary DNA (cDNA)	DNA that is identical to a native DNA containing a gene of interest except that the cDNA lacks non coding regions (introns) because it is synthesized in the laboratory using mRNA templates.
Conformation	The three dimensional arrangement of a molecule which depends upon the spatial orientation of its chemical bonds.
Conjugation	A recombination mechanism that results in the transfer of genetic material between two bacterial cells that are temporarily joined.
Contraception	The prevention of pregnancy.

Term	Definition
Convection	The mass movement of warmed air or liquid to or from the surface of a body or object.
Constitutive enzymes	Enzymes synthesized in fixed amounts independent of need.
Cori cycle	During vigorous exercise, pyruvate produced by glycolysis in muscle is converted to lactate-by-lactate dehydrogenase. The lactate diffuses into the blood stream and is carried to the liver. Here it is converted to glucose by gluconeogenesis. The glucose is released into the bloodstream and becomes available for uptake by muscle (as well as other tissues, including brain). This cycle of reactions is called the cori cycle. **Liver → Muscle →** Glucose → Glucose Gluconeogenesis → Blood → Pyruvate → PyruvateLactate → $NADH + H^+$ → Lactate $NADH + H^+$Dehydrogenase NAD^+ → dehydrogenase NAD^+ → Lactate → Lactate
Cortex	The region of the root between the stele and epidermis filled with growth tissue.
Cotyledons	The one (monocot) or two (dicot) seed leaves of an angiosperm embryo.
Coupled reactions	Two chemical reactions which have a common intermediate.
Covalent bond	A chemical bond formed between two atoms by the sharing of a pair of electrons.
Crude fiber	What remains of dietary fiber after acid and alkaline treatment? This consists of primary cellulose and lignin.
Cumulative effect	The action of two alleles of gene giving a more pronounced effect than one in the heterozygous condition.
Cytoplasm	The region of a cell inside the cell membrane and outside the nucleus; or the protoplasm of the cell surrounding the nucleus.
Cytoplasmic male sterility	A type of pollen sterility transmitted through the cytoplasm, maternally inherited.
Cytokinins	A class of related plant hormones that retard aging and act in concert with auxins to stimulate cell division influence the pathway of differentiation and control apical dominance.

Term	*Definition*
Cytokinesis	The division of the cytoplasm to form two separate daughter cells immediately after mitosis.
Cytosine	Nitrogen base one of two pyrimidines found in both DNA and RNA.
Cytosol	The cytosol is the soluble part of the cytoplasm where a large number of metabolic reactions take place.
Dalton	The atomic mass unit. A measure of mass for atoms and subatomic particles.
Dark reaction	That portion of the photosynthetic process, which does not require light. Chemical energy in the form of ATP and reduced ferrdoxin is produced from light energy in the light reaction, and this chemical energy is used to use to carry on biosynthesis in the dark reaction.
Denaturation	A process in which a protein unravels and loses its native conformation, thereby becoming biologically inactive. Denaturation occurs under extreme conditions of pH, salt concentration and temperature.
De novo synthesis	Refers to the complete synthesis of a substance from its ultimate precursors as opposed to the final steps in the synthesis.
Density	The number of individuals per unit area or volume.
Deoxyribonucleic acid (DNA)	A double-stranded helical nucleic acid molecule capable of replicating and determining the inherited structure of cell's proteins.
Determination	The progressive restriction of developmental potential, causing the possible fate of each cell to become more limited as the embryo develops.
Dextran	Dextran consists of glucose residues linked mainly by a1 6 bonds but with occasional branch points that may be formed by a 1 2, a 2 3 or a 1 4 bonds.
Dietary fiber	Substances in food (essentially from plants) that are not digested by the processes present in the stomach and small intestine.
Diffusion	The spontaneous tendency of a substance to move down its concentration gradient from a more concentrated to a less concentrated area.

Term	Definition
Digestion	The process of breaking down food into molecules small enough for the body to absorb.
Dihybrid	A hybrid for two different genes.
Diploid	Having a chromosome number just twice the haploid gametic number.
Disaccharide	A sugar, which yields two monomer sugar units (monosaccharides) on hydrolysis or two units of sugar united by glucosidic bond.
Dispersion	The distribution of individuals within geographical population boundaries.
DNA	The purine and pyrimidine bases of DNA carry genetic information whereas the sugar and phosphate groups perform a structural role.
DNA synthesis	Studies have shown that RNA synthesis is essential for the initiation of DNA synthesis. Furthermore, a short stretch of RNA is covalently linked to newly synthesized DNA fragments. Thus, RNA primes the synthesis of DNA. DNA RNA Protein transcription translation
DNA-DNA hybridization	The comparison of whole genomes of two species by estimating the extent of hydrogen bonding that occurs between single-stranded DNA obtained from the two species.
DNA-ligase	A linking enzyme essential for DNA replication catalyzes the covalent bonding of the 3′ end of a new DNA fragment of the 5′ end of a growing chain.
DNA-polymerase	An enzyme that catalyzes the elongation of new DNA at a replication fork in the 5′ 3′ direction by the addition of nucleotides to the existing chain.
DNA-probe	A chemically synthesized, radioactively labeled segment of nucleic acid used to find a gene of interest by hydrogen-bonding to a complementary sequence.
DNA sequence	The DNA sequence is the sequence of A, C, G, and T along the DNA molecule, which carries the genetic information.
DNA double helix	Ina DNA double helix, the two strand of DNA are wound round each other with the bases on the inside and the sugar-phosphate backbones on the outside. The two DNA

Term	*Definition*
	chains are held together by hydrogen bonds between pairs of bases; adenine (A) always pairs with thiamine (T) and guanine (G) always pairs with cytosine (C).
Domain	1. A structural and functional portion of a polypeptide that may be coded for by a specific exon; a globular region of a protein with tertiary structure. 2. A taxonomic category above the kingdom level; the three domains are archaebacteria, eubacteria and eukaryotes.
Dt gene maize	A "genic mutagen" in chromosome 9 in maize causing a (chromosome 3) to mutate to A, yielding dotted kernels or leaves streaked with anthocyanin.
Electrochemical gradient	The diffusion gradient of an ion, representing a type of potential energy that accounts for both the concentration difference of the ion across a membrane and its tendency to move relative to the membrane potential.
Electrogenic pump	An ion transport protein generating voltage across the membrane.
Electron carriers	NADH, NADPH, $FADPH_2$ are the major electron carrier or A substance which can gain or lose electrons reversibly and which participates in the transfer of electrons from one molecule to another.
Electron microscopy	A technique for visualizing material at very high magnification with resolutions attainable down to about 10 Å. Beams of electrons rather than light rays are employed.
Electron transport chain	The series of carriers responsible for transporting electrons from substrate to oxygen during respiration.
Endergonic process.	A process, which proceeds with an increase in free energy. It is not spontaneous and must be driven by coupling to some other process, which can supply energy.
Endocytosis	Endocytosis is the uptake of macromolecules from the extra cellular space into the cell across the plasma membrane via the formation of an intracellular vesicle pinching off from the plasma membrane.
Endoplasmic reticulum (ER)	An extensive membranous network in eukaryotic cells, continuous with the outer nuclear membrane and composed of ribosome-studded (rough) and ribosome-free (smooth) regions.

Term	Definition
Energy	The capacity to do work by moving matter against an opposing force.
Energy of fat	A gram of nearly anhydrous fat store more than six times as much energy as a gram of hydrated glycogen.
Energy production or consumption	$NADH + H^+ + \frac{1}{2} O_2$ $NAD^+ + H_2O DG° = -52.6$ Kcal/mol (exergonic), $DE° = + 1.14$ Volts ADP + Pi + H$^+$ ATP + H_2O DG° = +7.3 Kcal/mol (endergonic), $DE° = -30.5$ KJ/mol. ATP + H_2O ADP + Pi
Energy used	The synthesis of one molecule of glucose from two molecules of pyruvate requires six molecules of ATP.
Energy value	The span of the respiratory chain is 1.14 Volts, which is corresponds to 53 Kcal.
Energy yield	Two ATPs are used in glycolysis and four ATPs are synthesized for each molecule of glucose so that the net yield is two ATPs per glucose. Under aerobic conditions, the two NADH molecules arising from glycolysis also yield energy via oxidative phosphorylation.
Enzymes	Protein molecules, which are specific and efficient catalysts of certain chemical reactions; or a complex organic substance (a specific protein or biocatalyst) that accelerates (catalyzes) a specific chemical reaction; or protein catalysts called enzymes are mediators of the dynamic events of life; an enzyme catalyzes almost every chemical reaction in a cell.
Endergonic reaction	A no spontaneous chemical reaction in which free energy is absorbed from the surroundings.
Enhancer	A DNA sequence that recognizes certain transcription factors that can stimulate transcription of nearby genes.
Entropy	A quantitative measure of disorder or randomness, symbolized by S.
Epistatic gene	A gene, which suppresses the action of another gene not at the same locus in the chromosome.
Erythrocyte	A red blood cell contains hemoglobin, which functions in transporting oxygen in the circulatory system.
Equilibrium	A state in which there are no further changes in the properties of a system with time. For a chemical reaction this means that the concentrations of reactants and products do not change further with time.

Term	Definition
Equilibrium potential	The membrane potential for a given ion at which the voltage exactly balances the chemical diffusion gradient for that ion.
Essential amino acids (indispensable)	Amino acids not efficiently synthesized by humans that must therefore be included in the diet. There are eight amino acids.
Essential nutrient	1. A chemical element required for a plant to grow from a seed and complete the life cycle. 2. A nutrient substance that an animal cannot make itself from raw materials but that must be obtained in food in prefabricated form.
Ethylene	The only gaseous plant hormone, responsible for fruit ripening, growth inhibition, leaf abscission, and aging.
Eukaryotes	Eukaryotic cells have a membrane-bound nucleus and a number of other membrane-bound subcellular (internal) organelles, each of which has a specific function.
Evolution	The process by which gradual shifts in the nature of a living population leads, after many generations, to the appearance of new characteristics in the population.
Exergonic process	A process, which proceeds with a decrease in free energy. A spontaneous process.
Exergonic reaction	A spontaneous chemical reaction in which there is a net release of free energy.
Exocytosis	Exocytosis is the secretion of proteins out of the cell across the plasma membrane into the extra cellular space.
Exon	The coding region of a eukaryotic gene that is expressed. Exons are separated from each other by introns.
Exotoxin	A toxic protein secreted by a bacterial cell that produces specific symptoms even in the absence of the bacterium.
Fat	A biological compound consisting of three fatty acids linked to one glycerol molecule.
Fatty acid	A long carbon chain carboxylic acid. Fatty acids vary in length and in the number and location of double bonds; three fatty acids linked to a glycerol molecule from fat.
Faraday	The change in one mole of electrons to 96,500 coulombs.
Feedback inhibition	A method of metabolic control in which the end product of a metabolic pathway acts as an inhibitor of an enzyme within that pathway.

Term	Definition
Fermentation	The biochemical degradation of sugar and other food stuffs by reactions which take place under anaerobic conditions (i.e., in the absence of oxygen) or A catabolic process that makes a limited amount of ATP from glucose without an electron transport chain and that produces a characteristic end-product, such as ethyl alcohol or lactic acid.
Fertility restorers	Cytoplasmic male sterile lines will produce viable pollen in certain genotypes. Restorers have genes that restore fertility to a cytoplasmic male sterile line.
Fertilization	The union of haploid gametes to produce a diploid zygote.
Flavoprotein	A protein molecule, which contains flavin adenine dinucleotide (FAD) or flavin mononucleotide (FMN) as a prosthetic group. The flavoprotiens are involved in many oxidation-reduction reactions in the cell.
F_1 generation	The first filial or hybrid offspring in a genetic cross-fertilization.
F_2 generation	Offspring resulting from interbreeding of the hybrid F_1 generation.
Fiber	A lignified cell type that reinforces the xylem of angiosperms and functions in mechanical support, a slender, tapered sclerenchyma cell that usually occurs in bundles.
First law of thermodynamics	The principle of conservation of energy. Energy can be transferred and transformed but it cannot be created or destroyed.
Free energy change	A measure of the maximum useful work it is possible to obtain from a process carried out at constant temperature and pressure.
Free radical	Short lived form of compounds that exist with an unpaired electron in their outer electron shell. This causes it to have an electron-seeking nature, which can be very destructive to electron-dense areas of a cell, such as DNA and cell membranes.
Galactoside	A molecule containing galactose in which some group other than hydrogen is attached to the hydroxyl group at the C-1 atom of galactose. The prefix a or b refers to the orientation of this group above or below the galactose ring.

Term	Definition
G$_1$ phase	The first growth phase of the cell cycle, consisting portion of interphase before DNA synthesis begins.
G$_2$ phase	The second growth phase of the cell cycle, consisting portion of interphase after DNA synthesis occurs.
Gel-electrophoresis	Separation of nucleic acids or proteins on the basis of their size and electric charge by measuring their rate of movement through an electric field in a gel.
Gene	The unit of heredity. The factor controlling a hereditary trait; or One of many discrete units of hereditary information located on the chromosomes and consisting of DNA or the discrete particulate hereditary determiner located in the chromosome in linear order; the 'element' of Mendel and factor of early genetic terminology.
Gene amplification	The selective synthesis of DNA, which results in multiple copies of a single gene, thereby enhancing expression.
Gene cloning	Formation by a bacterium, carrying foreign genes in a recombinant plasmid of a clone of identical cells containing the replicated foreign genes.
Gene organization	Most protein-coding genes in eukaryotes consist of coding sequences called exons, interrupted by non coding sequences called introns.
Genetics	The science of heredity of similarities and differences among organisms.
Generally recognized as safe (GRAS)	A group of food additives that in 1958 were considered safe, therefore allowing manufactures to use them thereafter when needed in food products.
Genetic code	The genetic code is the relationship between the sequence of bases in DNA (or its RNA transcripts) and the sequence of amino acids in proteins.
Genetic code is a triplet code	The genetic code is the set of rules that specify how the nucleotide sequence of an mRNA is translated into the amino acid sequence of a polypeptide. The nucleotide sequence is read as triplets called codons. The codons UAG, UGA, and UAA do not specify an amino acid and are called termination codons or stop codons. AUG codes for methionine and also acts as an initiation or start codon.

Term	Definition
Genetic engineering	Alteration of genetic material in plants or animals with the intent of improving growth, disease resistance or other characteristics.
Genome	A set of chromosomes (n) inherited as unit.
Genomic clone	A selected host cell with a vector containing a fragment of genomic DNA from a different organism.
Genomic library	A set of thousand of DNA segments from a genome each carried by a plasmid or phase.
Genotype	The genetic constitution or gene makeup of an organism.
Germplasm	A special kind of protoplasm transmitted unchanged from generation to generation.
Gibberellins	A class of related plant hormones that stimulate growth in the stem and leaves, trigger germination of seeds and breaking of bud dormancy and stimulate fruit development with auxin.
Glycemic Index	A ratio used to measure the relative ability of a carbohydrate to raise blood glucose levels as opposed to the ability of white bread/glucose to raise blood glucose levels.
Glycogen	A polypeptide hormone that is secreted by the α-cells of the pancreas when the blood sugar level is low. This hormone increases the blood sugar level by stimulating the breakdown of glycogen in the liver.
Glycogen metabolism	Glycogen degradation and glycogen synthesis are controlled both by allosteric regulation and by hormonal control.
Glycolysis	This set of biochemical reactions in which glucose or the glucose polymer glycogen is converted into lactic acid.
Gluconeogenesis	Gluconeogenesis synthesizes glucose from non-carbohydrate precursors and is important for the maintenance of blood glucose levels during starvation or during vigorous exercise. The brain and erythrocytes depend almost entirely on blood glucose as an energy source. Gluconeogenesis occurs mainly in the liver and to a lesser extent in the kidney. Most enzymes of gluconeogenesis are cytosolic, but pyruvate carboxylase and glucose-6-phosphate are located in the mitochondrial matrix and bound to the smooth endoplasmic reticulum respectively.

Term	Definition
Glycolysis	The set of biochemical reactions in which glucose or the glucose polymer glycogen is converted into lactic acid.
Gonad	A gland such as an ovary or testis in which gametes are produced.
Gout	A metabolic disease marked by an excess of uric acid in the blood accompanied by painful inflammation of the joints.
Green house effect	The warming of the earth due to atmospheric accumulation of carbon dioxide, which absorbs infrared radiation and slows its escape from the irradiated earth.
Growth	An increase in the size or number of cells representing a net increase in total cellular matter.
Guanine	A nitrogen base one of two purine found in both DNA and RNA.
Half-cell reaction	A chemical reaction, which describes a substance gaining or losing electrons and which therefore, describes one half of an oxidation-reduction reaction.
Haploid	Having half the number of chromosomes found in diploid organisms.
Hardy-Weinberg law	A law concerning gene frequencies in populations. It states that after one generation of random mating gene frequencies remain constant in future generations.
Heredity	The transmission of genes and there by traits controlled by these genes from parent to offspring.
Heritability	The extent to which a given trait is determined by inheritance.
Heteroploid	Having a chromosome number differing from the normal number.
Heterosis	Hybrid vigour a term coined by George H. Shull.
Histones	Histones play a role in the packing of DNA molecules, rendering them more compact. Some of the nonhistone proteins associated with chromosomes are more likely participants in the specific control of gene function.

Term	Definition
HIV	Human immunodeficiency virus. The infections agent that causes AIDS; HIV is an RNA retrovirus. AID; (Acquired immunodeficiency syndrome) The name of the late stages of HIV infection; defined by a specified reduction of T cells and the appearance of characteristic secondary infections.
Homologous chromosomes	Chromosomes which pair at meiotic prophase and are similar in size, shape, structure and function. They have alleles of the same genes.
Hormone	A chemical substance produced by one tissue in an organism, which exerts some controlling influence on other tissues in the same organism; or One of many types of circulating chemical signals in all multicellular organisms that are formed in specialized cells, travel in body fluids and coordinate the various parts of the organism by interacting with target cells.
Host cell	A cell (usually a bacterium) in which a vector can be propagated.
Hybrid	A cross of unlike organisms.
Hybridization	The process of making a hybrid by cross-pollination in plants or by mating two types of animals.
Hydrogen bond	A weak attractive force between a hydrogen atom and a second atom. Such bonds are generally formed only if the second atom is very electronegative (such as N, O or Cl) and the hydrogen atom is also covalently bound to an electronegative atom.
Hydrophilic	Having an affinity for water
Hydrophobic	Having an aversion to water, tending to coalesce and form droplets in water.
Hydrophobic interactions	Nonpolar molecules contain neither ions nor dipolar bonds and thus these molecules do not become hydrated. Because they are insoluble or almost insoluble in water they are called hydrophobic.
Hyperglycemia	High blood glucose levels above 140 milligrams per 100 ml of blood.
Hypoglycemia	Low blood glucose levels, below 40 to 50 mg/100 ml of blood.
Hypostatic gene	A gene whose phenotypic effects are suppressed by another gene not at the same locus in the chromosome.

Term	Definition
Hydrolysis	The cleavage of a chemical bond by reaction with water.
Induced chromosome break	Chromosome break caused by some agent usually external to the chromosome, such as radiation or chemicals.
In Situ **hybridization**	For in situ hybridization a tissue sample is incubated with a labeled nucleic acid probe, excess probe is washed away and the location of hybridized probe is examined. The technique enables the spatial localization of gene expression to be determined as well as the location of individual genes on chromosomes.
Inhibitor	A substance, which lowers the rate of a chemical reaction. (Some times called a negative catalyst)
Initial velocity	The rate of a chemical reaction at zero time when essentially no reactant has been converted to product.
Insulin	The vertebrate hormone that lowers blood sugar levels by promoting the uptake of glucose by most body cells and promoting the synthesis and storage of glycogen in the liver; also stimulates protein and fat synthesis; secreted by endoplasmic cells of the pancreas called is lets of Lange Hans.
Inversion in genetics	A rearrangement of a chromosome in which a portion is rotated a full 180 degrees. It sometimes results when a chromosome is broken at two places.
Ion	An atom with an unequal number of electrons and protons. If the number of electrons exceeds the number of protons, the ion is negative. If the number of protons exceeds the number of electrons the ion is positive.
Ionizing radiation	Any of the high-energy radiations that displace electrons from neutral atoms.
Isoelectric focusing	In isoelectric focusing, proteins are separated by electrophoresis in a pH gradient in a gel. They separate on the basis of their relative content of positively and negatively charged residues. Each protein migrates through the gel unit it reaches the point where it has no net charge, its isoelectric point (PI).
Isoenzymes	Isoenzymes are different forms of an enzyme, which catalyze the same reaction, but which exhibit different physical or kinetic properties.

Term	Definition
Isomer	Different chemical structures for compounds that share the same chemical formula or one of several organic compounds with the same molecular formula but different structures and therefore different properties. The three types are structural isomers, geometric isomers and optional isomers.
Isotope	An alternate form of a chemical element. It differs from other atoms of the same element in the number of neutrons in its nucleus.
Karyotype	The character of the chromosomal complement with reference to the comparative size, shape and morphology of the different chromosomes.
Kinetic energy	It is the energy of movement the motion of a car, for example, or the motion of molecules.
Law of independent assortment	Mendel's second law, stating that each allele pair segregates independently during gamete formation; applies when gene for two traits are located on different pairs of homologous chromosomes.
Law of segregation	Mendel's first law, stating that allele pairs separate during gamete formation and then randomly reform pairs during the fusion of gametes at fertilization.
Lecithin	A group of phospholipids containing two fatty acids a phosphate group and a choline molecules.
Library (genomic)	A complete set of genomic clones from an organism or of cDNA clones from one cell type.
Ligand	A molecule that binds specifically to a macromolecule (other than the substrate or products of an enzyme) is often called a ligand of that macromolecule.
Light reaction	That potion of the photosynthetic process in which light energy is converted into chemical energy.
Lignin	An insoluble fiber made up of a multiringed alcohol structure.
Limiting amino acid	The essential amino acid in the lowest concentration in a food in comparison with the body's need.
Lipid	One of a family of compounds including fats, phospholipids, and steroids that are insoluble in water.

Term	Definition
Locus	The physical location of a gene in the chromosome.
Low input sustainable agriculture(LISA)	A from of farming that attempts to limit use of purchased materials such as manufactured fertilizers and pesticides. Use of manure and crop rotaion is typical substitutes.
Lysis	Destruction of a bacterium as by bacteriophase, with the multiplication of phase particles in the process.
Meiosis	A two stage type of cell division in sexually reproducing organisms that results in gametes with half the chromosome number of the original cell; or a special type of cell division found in gamete production. It consists of two divisions, one of which is reductional. Homologous chromosomes pair and assort at random to produce gametes with the haploid number chromosomes.
Melanin	A black or brown pigment of animal origin. In albinos a mutant recessive gene blocks the production of melanin.
Mendelian population	A naturally breeding unit, isolated by some mechanism from other units of sexually reproducing plants or animals.
Membrane	A selectively permeable boundary surrounding the cell or surrounding various subcellular particles.
Mendel's law	The principle that hereditary characters are determined by discrete particles (genes) that segregates at random in gamete formation.
Metabolism	The sum of all the chemical process occurring in a cell.
Metaphase	The stage in the cell division at which the chromosomes are shortened and arranged on an equatorial plate in the center of the cell.
Microspore	The "small spore" an asexual spore, the pollen grain in plants, in which develop the male gametes, the sperm.
Michaelis constant	The constant, km, derived from the Michaelis Menten equation, which expresses the substrate concentration necessary to produce one-half of the maximum velocity in an enzymatic reaction.
Michaelis-Menten model	$E + S \underset{}{\overset{K1}{\rightleftharpoons}} ES \xrightarrow{K3} E + P$

Term	Definition
Michaelis-Menten equation	$K_2 V_{max} [S] Vo = km + [S]$
Michaelis constant	$Km = K_2 + K_3 Km = K_1$
Micron (μ)	A unit of length equal to 10^{-4} cm.
Microsomes	A subcellular particulate fraction usually containing ribosome and endoplasmic reticulum. Experimentally, it is the material sedimenting in an ultracentrifuge at a force of bout 100,000 × gravity.
Mitosis	A process of cell division in eukaryotic cells conventionally divided into the growth period (inter phase) and four stages: prophase, metaphase, anaphase and telophase. The stages conserve chromosome number by equally allocating replicated chromosome to each of the daughter cells.
Monoecious	Having male and female reproductive organs in the same individual.
Monosaccaride	Only one unit of sugar, e.g., glucose, fructose, mannose.
Monosomic	Having a full set of chromosome minus one chromosome, $2n - 1$.
Morphology	The study or science of structure at any level of organization (sub-cellular, cellular, tissue, organ or gross structure of organisms).
Mitochondria	Membrane-surrounded structures, which contain the respiratory enzyme systems and electron transport chain. Mitochondria are found in the cytoplasm of cells.
Multiple alleles	More than the normal two alleles at a locus in the chromosome.
Mutable gene	An unstable gene that mutates frequently.
Mutant	A variant from the normal or wild type that is inherited in a Mendelian manner.
Mutator gene	A gene that causes other genes to mutate, e.g., Dt. In corn causes a to change to A.
Muton	A subdivision of the gene, the smallest element, alteration of which can be effective in causing a mutation.
Nearest-neighbour frequency	In nucleic acid structure, the relative number of times each of the four nucleotides is found adjacent to any given nucleotide.

Term	Definition
Negative control of gene transcription	Negative control of transcription is the situation when a bound repressor protein prevents transcription of structural genes.
Nitrogen fixation	The assimilation of atmospheric nitrogen by certain prokaryotic in to nitrogenous compounds that can be directly used by plants.
Non-polar molecule	A molecule in which the electrons are evenly distributed over the structure in such a fashion that there is no separation of charge.
Northern blotting	Northern blotting is analogous to southern blotting except that the sample nucleic acid that is separated by gel electrophoresis in RNA rather than DNA.
Nucleic acid	A biological molecule (such as RNA or DNA) that allows organisms to reproduce; polymers compound of monomers called nucleotides joined by covalent bonds (phosphodiester linkages) between the phosphate of one nucleotide and the sugar of the next nucleotide.
Nucleoside	A hydrolytic product of nucleic acids containing a heterocyclic nitrogen base attached to a pentose, generally ribose or deoxyribose.
Nucleotide	A phosphate ester derivative of a nucleoside.
Nucleus	The nucleus is a store of the cell's genetic information such as DNA in Chromosomes.
Nullisonic	The complete lack of a given chromosome pair; $2n - 2$.
Nutrients	Chemical substances in food that nourish the body by providing energy, building materials and factors to regulate needed chemical reactions in the body.
Nutrition	The council on food and nutrition of the American Medical Association defines nutrition as "the science of food; the nutrients and the substances therein; their action, interaction and balance in relation to health and diseases and the process by which the organism (i.e., body) ingests, digest, absorbs, transports, utilizes and excretes food substances".

Term	Definition
Okazaki fragments	DNA synthesis proceeds in a 5' → 3' direction on each strand of the parental DNA. On the strand with 3' → 5' orientation (the leading strand) the new DNA is synthesized continuously. On the strand that has 5' → 3' orientation (the lagging strand) the DNA is synthesized discontinuously as series of short okazaki fragments that are then joined together. The small fragments are called Okazaki fragments. The new DNA strand, which is made by this discontinuous method, is called the lagging strand.
Oligonucleotide	A group of several nucleotides bound together in phosphodiester linkage between the phosphate of one nucleotide and a hyderoxyl group on the sugar of an adjacent nucleotide.
Omega-3 (ω-3) fatty acid	A fatty acid with itsfirst double bond first appearing at the thrid carbon atom from the methyl end ($-CH_3$).
Operon	An operon is a coordinated unit of genetic expression.
Out breeding	Mating of unrelated individuals or of individuals not closely related; the opposite of inbreeding.
Ovary	The female reproductive organ in which eggs are produced. In plants, the overy, containing ovules is at the base of the pistil.
Over dominance	An effect in the heterozygote, A/a greater than in the homozygous dominant, A/A.
Ovule	The megasporangium of a seed palnt. After fertilization it becomes the seed.
Oxidation	A chemical change involving a loss of electrons.
Oxidative phosphorylation	Oxidative phosphorylation is ATP synthesis linked to the oxidation of NADH and $FADH_2$ by electron transport through the respiratory chain. Approximately three ATP molecules are synthesized per NADH oxidized and approximately two ATPs are synthesized per $FADH_2$ oxidized.
Oxidizing agent	In one sense, a substance capable of capturing an electron from another compound.
Paracentric inversion	A rotation of a segment of chromosome a full 180°, with the centromere beyond inversion, which is all within one arm of chromosome.

Term	Definition
Parmutation	A mutation in which one allele in heterozygous condition changes permanently its partner allele.
Parthenogenesis	Reproduction without fertilization.
Passive transport	The movement of molecules across a membrane by passive transport does not require an input of metabolic energy. The molecule moves from a high concentration to a lower concentration, e.g. transportation of water, gases and urea.
Pedigree	The genotype of an individual; a chart showing the ancestral history of an individual.
Pericarp	The outer layers of cells surrounding the seed.
PH	The negative logarithm of the hydrogen ion concentration.
Phagocytosis	Phagocytosis is the uptake of large particles (bacteria and cell debris). The particle binds to receptors on the surface of the phagocytic cell and the plasma membrane then engulfs the particle and ingests it via the formation of large endocytic vesicle, a phagosome.
Phenotype	The appearance of an individual produced by the genotype in co-operation with the environment.
Phenylketonuria	A disease inflicting serious brain damage in infants, caused by a recessive gene. It renders a child unable to metabolize phenylpyruvic acid, which accumulates in the brain.
Photoperiodism	The action of certain amounts of light stimulating floral initiation in plants.
Photo-Phosphorylation	The process of generating ATP from ADP and phosphate by means of a proton-motive force generated by the thylakoid membrane of the chloroplast during the light reactions of photosynthesis.
Photo respiration	A metabolic pathway that consumes oxygen, evolves carbon dioxide, generates no ATP, and decreases photosynthetic out put; generally occurs on hot, dry, bright days, when stomata close and the oxygen concentration in the leaf exceeds that close of carbon dioxide.

Term	Definition
Phototropism	Growth of a plant shoot toward or away from light.
Photosynthesis	The conversion of light energy into chemical energy and the use of that energy to form carbohydrate and other cellular constituents from carbon dioxide and water. OR Photosynthesis is a chemical process it uses solar energy to synthesize carbohydrate from carbon dioxide and water. In the light reactions, the light energy derives the synthesis of NADPH and ATP. In the dark reactions (carbon-fixation reactions), the NADPH and ATP are used to synthesize carbohydrate from CO_2 and H_2O.
Pinocytosis	Pinocytosis is the non specific uptake of extracellular fluid via small endoplastic vesicles that pinch off from the plasma membrane. This is a constitutive process occurring in all eukaryotic cells.
Pistil	The ovule-bearing organ of a flower at the base of the style.
Pistillate	Bearing female gametes only have a female type with no stamens.
Plant Biochemistry	It deals with chemical manifestation of plant metabolism. Plant biochemist interested in studying properties of plant kingdom e.g. Photosynthesis, chlorophyll synthesis, energy biosynthesis and chemical compounds biosynthesis.
Plasmagene	A unit in the cytoplasm causing hereditary traits, e.g., kappa in paramecium.
Plasmid	A small ring of DNA that carries accessory genes separate from those of a bacterial chromosome.
Plastids	Small bodies of specialized protoplasm, especially in plant cells, e.g., chloroplasts containing the green pigment chlorophyll.
Pollen grain	The microspore in plants containing a tube nucleus and a generative nucleus that divides either in pollen grain or in pollen tube to form two sperm nuclei.
Pollen parent (male parent)	The plant supplying the pollen for a hybrid.
Polymers	Polymers are composed of many copies of a few small molecules linked in chains by covalent bonds. These subunits of polymers are referred to as monomers or residues.

Term	Definition
Poly gene	One of many genes necessary for a given phenotypic effect as found in quantitative inheritance.
Polypeptides	Polypeptides are polymers composed of amino acids connected by peptide bonds. It can be described in four groups: 1. Primary structure, 2. Secondary structure, 3. Tertiary structure, and 4. Quaternary structure.
Polyploid	Composed of more than two genomes or chromosome sets. 2n = diploid, 3n = triploid, 4n = tetraploid etc.
Polysaccharide	A polymeric sugar yielding many monosaccharide units upon hydrolysis; or at least 15 different sugars are used to form various polysaccharides. The monomeric sugars can be bonded to one another in multiple ways; thus, many polysaccharides are nonlinear; branched molecules.
Population genetics	The branch of genetics concerned with the frequencies of genes (alleles) in a population.
Positive control of gene transcription	Positive control of gene transcription is when the regulatory protein (an activator) binds to DNA and turns on transcription.
Potential energy	The energy that usually concerns us when we study biological or chemical systems is potential energy or stored energy.
Probability	The chance or likelihood of a given possible event.
Prophase	A stage of cell division in which chromosomes are first visible as chromosomes.
Prototroph	A wild type bacterium that will grow on a minimal medium.
Protein	A three dimensional biological polymer constructed from a set of 20 different monomers called amino acids; or proteins are synthesized in the amino-to-carboxyl direction by the sequential addition of amino acids to the carboxyl end of the growing peptide chain.
Proton pump	An active transport mechanism in cell membranes that consumes ATP to force hydrogen ions out of a cell and in the process generates a membrane potential.
Primary structure of protein	The linear sequence of amino acids joined together by peptide bonds is termed the primary structure of the protein.

Term	Definition
Prokaryotes	Prokaryotes (bacteria and blue-green algae) are the most abundant organisms on earth. A prokaryotic cell does not contain a membrane-bound nucleus.
Protamines	In sperm heads, DNA is particularly highly condensed and here the histones are replaced with small basic proteins called protamines.
Purine	One of two families of nitrogenous bases found in nucleotides consisting of two members: adenine (A) and guanine (G).
Pyrimidine	One of two families of nitrogenous bases found in nucleotides consisting of three members: cytosine (C), thymine (T) and uracil (U).
Pyridine nucleotide	Both nicotinamide adenine dinucleotide (NAD^+) and nicotiamine adenine dinucleotide phosphate ($NADP^+$).
Quaternary structure of protein	If a protein is made up of more than one polypeptide chain it is said to have quaternary structure. This refers to the spatial arrangement of the polypeptide subunits and the nature of interactions between them.
Radioactive	Having a nucleus that gives off particles and energy; characteristic of unstable isotopes of a chemical element.
Rate constant	Proportionality constant between the rates of a reaction on the concentration of species, which influence the rate.
Rate law	An equation expressing the dependence of the rate of a reaction on the concentration of species, which influence the rate.
Recessive	A term coined by Mendel to describe characters, which recede completely in the F_1. Action of the recessive allele is suppressed by the dominant.
Reciprocal crosses	Hybrids made by using the mutant type as female in one case and as male in the other.
Recombination	A new combination of linked genes other than the parental types, e.g., in an F_1 of AB/ab genotype. Both Ab and aB gametes would represent recombination.
Redox potential	The oxidation-reduction potential, E, (or redox potential) of a substance is a measure of its affinity for electrons. The standard redox potential (E'_0) is measured under standard conditions, at pH 7.0 and is expressed in volts.

Term	Definition
Reduction	The gaining of electrons by a substance involved in a redox reaction.
Repressible enzymes	Enzymes whose rate of production is decreased when the intracellular concentration of certain metabolites increases.
Respiration	The oxidative breakdown and releases of energy from fuel molecules by reaction with oxygen in aerobic cells.
Respiratory control	The control of respiration by limiting levels of the acceptor molecule ADP.
Respiratory quotient (RQ)	Moles of CO_2 producedMoles of O_2 consume.
Restriction enzyme	Restriction enzymes allow DNA to be cut at specific sites, nucleic acid hybridization allows the detection of specific nucleic acid sequences, DNA sequencing can be used to easily determine the nucleotide sequence of a DNA molecule; or A degradative enzyme that recognizes and cuts up DNA (including that of certain phases) that is foreign to a cell.
Restriction fragment lengthpoymorphisms (RFLPs)	Differences in DNA sequence on homologous chromosomes that result in different patterns of restriction fragment lengths (DNA segments resulting from treatment with restriction enzymes); useful as genetic markers for making linkage maps.
Reverse mutations	Mutations from a mutant type to the normal or wild type allele. Less frequent than the mutation from the wild type to the mutant.
Reversible process	A process occurring so slowly in a system that the system is at all times in a state of equilibrium. The process can be stopped and reversed just by making an infinitesimal change in the external conditions.
Ribosome	A cytoplasmic nucleoprotein particle, consisting of RNA and protein. Ribosomes are the site of protein synthesis.

Term	Definition
RNA synthesis	RNA synthesis differs from that of DNA in several ways. RNA polymerase does not require a primer. The DNA template is fully conserved in RNA synthesis. Whereas it is semi conserved in DNA synthesis. RNA polymerase has no known nuclease activities. The growth of an RNA chain is in the 5′ → 3′ direction as in DNA synthesis. RNA polymerase moves along the DNA template strand in the 3′ → 5′ direction, since the DNA template strand is anti-parallel to the newly synthesized RNA strand. The sequence of long RNA chains can be elucidated by the use of specific hydrolytic enzymes and finger printing methods.
Second law of thermodynamics	The principle where by every energy transfer or transformation increases the entropy of the universe. Ordered forms of energy are at least partly converted to heat and in spontaneous reactions, the free energy of the system also decreases.
Seed	The mature ovule containing a dormant plant embryo.
Self-fertilization	Fertilization following application of plants own pollen.
Self-pollination	Pollinating a plant with its own pollen; selfing.
Self-sterility	In capability of producing seed when self-pollinated. Several alleles, S_1, S_2, S_3 etc. are responsible for this phenomenon.
Self-tolerance	Cells that produce antibody that reacts with normal body components are killed early in fetal life so that the adult animal normally is unable to make antibodies against self, a condition called self-tolerance.
Secondary structure of protein	It refers to the regular folding of regions of the polypeptide chain (α-helix and β-plated sheet).
Sickle cell anemia	A condition produced by an abnormal hemoglobin molecule in the homo zygous condition.
Sickle cell trait	Trait shown by individuals characterized as heterozygote for the sickle cell gene.
Single cross	The hybrid of two pure lines.
Somatic cell	A cell in the body of the organism, with 2n chromosomes. The contrasting type is the germ cell, with n chromosomes.
Somatic mutation	A mutation in a somatic cell.

Term	Definition
Southern blotting	Southern blotting involves electrophoresis of DNA molecules in an agarose gel and then blotting the separated DNA bands on to a nitrocellulose filter. The filter is then incubated with a labeled DNA probe to detect those separated DNA bands that contain sequences complementary to the probe.
Spermatogenesis	Formation of mature sperm in animals.
Sporogenesis	The formation of microspores (pollen) and megaspores (embryo sac) in plants.
Sport	A mutation
Stages of cell division	1. Interphase, 2. Prophase, 3. Metaphase, 4. Anaphase and 5. Telophase.
Standard free energy change	The free energy change of a chemical process by which reactants at unit activity are converted into products at unit activity.
Staminate	Producing stamens only of a male plant.
Starch	Starch is a mixture of unbranched amylose (glucose residues joined by α, $1 \rightarrow 4$ bonds) and branched amylopectin (glucose residues joined α, $1 \rightarrow 4$ with some α, $1 \rightarrow 6$ branch points). Starch is produced in the stroma of chloroplasts and stored there as starch grains. Starch synthesis occurs from ADP-glucose, CDP-glucose or GDP-glucose (but not UDP-glucose).
State functions	Properties of the state of a system, which developed only upon the condition of a system and not its previous history.
Steady state	For an intermediate in a chemical reaction, a state in which the rate of breakdown of the intermediate is equal to the rate of its formation, with the result that its concentration does not change.
Stereoisomers	The D and L sterioisomers of sugars refers to the configuration of the asymmetric carbon atom furthest from the aldehyde or ketone group. The sugar is said to be a D isomer if the configuration of the atoms bonded to this carbon atom is the same as for the asymmetric carbon in D-glyceraldehydes.

Term	Definition
Stereo isomers	Substances which have the same molecular formula and order of attachment of atoms in the molecule but which differ in the three-dimensional geometry or configuration of the atoms.
Sterility	Inability to produce offspring.
Stigma	The upper end of the pistil that receives the pollen.
Substrate	The substrate whose reaction is catalyzed by an enzyme; or the chemicals that undergo a change in a reaction catalyzed by an enzyme are called substrate of that enzyme.
Sugar derivatives	Other groups to form a wide range of biologically important molecules including phosphorylated sugars, amino sugars and nucleotides can replace the hydroxyl groups of sugars.
Superoxide dismutase	An enzyme that can neutralize a superoxide free radical.
Suppressor	One, which suppresses the action of another gene or other genes.
Symbiosis	An ecological relationship between organisms of two different species that live together in direct contact.
Synthesis of palmitate	It requires the input of 8 molecules of acetyl CoA, 14 NADPH and 7 ATP.
Synapses	The conjugation or pairing of homologous chromosomes at meiosis.
Syndrome	A group of symptoms that occur together and characterize a disease.
Telophase	The last stage in cell division, in which the chromosomes are assembled at each end of the cell.
Template	A macromolecular mold for the synthesis of another macromolecule.
Terminalization	The movement of a chiasma away from the Centro mere and towards the end of a tetrad.
Tertiary structure of protein	Tertiary structure in a protein refers to the three-dimensional arrangement of all the amino acids in the polypeptide chain.

Term	Definition
Testcross	The cross of an F_1 by the homozygous recessive, useful in linkage studies. Contrast with backcross.
Tetrad	The group of four chromatids the results from pairing of homologous chromosomes and division of each chromosome into two chromatids.
Tetraploid	Having four genomes (4n) instead of two as in a diploid.
Threshold	A term used in studying effects of radiation. Below a certain dose, if there is a threshold, there is no measurable effect. No threshold exists for most genetic effects.
Three phases of transcription	Initiation → Elongation → Termination
Ti plasmid	A plasmid of a tumor-inducing bacterium that integrates a segment of its DNA into the host chromosome of aplant.
Tissue	An aggregate of cell of similar structure performing similar functions.
Transduction	The transfer of genes for bacterial characters by means of a phase particle acting as a messenger boy.
Transgenic organism	An organism containing certain genes from another species, produced for example by injecting foreign DAN into the nuclei of egg cells or early embryos.
Transformation	The heritable modification of the properties of one bacterial strain by an extract derived from cells of another strain; or the changing of the genotype of a micro-organism by combining with a transforming principle supplied; this principle is DNA.
Translocation	The exchange of parts of two nonhomologus chromosomes, following breakage either spontaneous or induced.
Trihybrid	A hybrid involving three gene pairs such as A/a, B/b, C/c and the offspring from such a hybrid.
Triploid	Having three genomes or sets of chromosomes (3n).
Turner's syndrome	An abnormality in human beings; individuals are phenotypically females, but have rudimentary sexual organs and mammary glands. Such individuals have but one X chromosome and no Y with a total of 45 chromosomes instead of the normal 46.

Term	Definition
Uracil	A nitrogen base, one of two pyrimidines found in RNA, but not DNA.
Uric acid	Uric acid, the major nitrogenous waste product of uricotelic organisms, is also formed in other organisms from the breakdown of purine bases. Gout is caused by the deposition of excess uric acid crystals in the joints.
Van der Waals Interactions	When two atoms approach one another closely, they create a nonspecific weak attractive force that produces a Van der Waals interaction.
Variegation	Diversity in characters in the same organism, e.g., alternating patches of green and white in leaves of some plants.
Vector	A plasmid or a viral DNA molecule in to which either a cDNA sequence or a genomic DNA sequence is inserted.
Virulent phase	A virus that kills the host bacterium. The contrasting type is temperate phase.
Virus	A small infectious agent required a host cell in which to reproduce. Its principal structure consists of DNA or RNA surrounded by a coat of protein; or A parasitic particle in plants and animals, some times causing disease, incapable of reproduction outside of the host cell.
Vitamin	An organic molecule required in the diet in very small amounts; vitamins serve primarily as coenzymes or parts of coenzymes.
Xanthophylls	A yellow-coloured compound $C_{40} H_{56} O_2$ found in plants.
X_0 condition	Having an X chromosome but no Y chromosome, as the female in poultry and same other birds.
Zymogen	An inactive precursor form of an enzyme.
Zwitterions	Amino acids in solution at neutral pH are pre-dominantly dipolar ions rather than un-ionized molecules are called zwitterions.
Zygote	The result of the fusion of male and female gametes; the individual that develops from such a fusion, usually diploid with 2n chromosomes.
Zygotic lethal	A lethal gene whose effect is in the embryo, larva or adult in contrast to the gametic lethal affecting a gamete.

4

TERMINOLOGY

Term	Explanation(s)
Acetaldehyde	An aldehyde formed from the oxidation of ethanol. An aldehyde contains a carbonyl group having only one hydrogen attached (formaldehyde, $H_2C=O$, is an exception).
Acetone	One of the ketone bodies that is present normally in the blood in small amounts but rises to toxic levels when there is not enough oxaloacetate to keep the TCA cycle functioning.
Acetyl-CoA	A two-carbon (acetyl) molecule made active by the attachment of coenzyme A. Acetyl-CoA is in a key position in the reclaiming of energy from fuel nutrients or in the synthesis of lipids derived from the consumption of excess fuel nutrients.
Acid-base balance	An optimal balance between the number of acidic ions and basic ions in the fluid of a tissue. This is a requirement for the continuation of life process since vital reactions can take place only when the pH is maintained within narrow limits. Both the respiratory and renal systems contribute to the maintenance of the acid-base balance by excreting or conserving the acidic or basic ions under their control.
Acidic amino acids	Amino acids whose side chains have an extra carboxyl (–COOH) group.
Acidosis	A set of conditions that would tend to lower the pH of blood if the body did not act to resist this change. Metabolic acidosis refers to changes in the bicarbonate concentration of the plasma; respiratory acidosis refers to changes in the carbon dioxide pressure.

Term	Explanation(s)
Active transport	Energy requiring transport of a solute across a membrane in the direction of greater concentration or in other words, against a concentration gradient. The usual, unassisted movement of molecules is by diffusion from a place of higher concentration to a place of lower concentration. The work of active transport to maintain concentration gradient in the cells of a human at rest is so great that it may consume as much as 30-40 per cent of the total input of energy.
Acyl carrier protein	A protein that has acid as its prosthetic group. It is active in the synthesis of fatty acids as it carries acyl groups that are bound to the pentothenic acid in a thioester linkage.
Aerobic reaction	A chemical reaction requiring oxygen.
Albinism	A rare recessive disorder in which the enzyme tyrosinase is missing in the pigmented cells.
Albumin	A serum globular protein that occurs in the highest concentration of the major serum protein.
Alcohol	A hydrocarbon in which a hydroxyl group has replaced one or more of the hydrogen.
Aliphatic	Belonging to that series of organic compounds characterized by open chains of carbon atoms rather than by rings.
Alkalosis	A set of conditions that would tend to raise the pH of the blood if the body did not act to resist this change.
Amino acid pool	The free amino acids present mainly in the cytosol and circulating blood. These amino acids may have joined the pool during either the digestion and absorption of protein rich foods or the degradation of body proteins. The amino acids stand ready to be incorporated into protein or used for fuel.
Ammonotelic	Organisms that excrete nitrogen as ammonia.
Anabolism	The energy requiring production of macromolecules from smaller molecules.
Anaerobic reaction	A chemical process that does not require oxygen.
Analbuminemia	A deficiency in the livers capacity to synthesize the protein albumin thus leading to a decrease in the plasma albumin.

Term	Explanation(s)
Antibody	A serum protein that is synthesized in response to the entry of a foreign substance (antigen).
Anticodon	A sequence of three bases in transfer RNA that is complementary to a sequence of three bases in messenger RNA.
Antimetabolite	A substance that bears a structural resemblance to a normal substrate or enzyme and thus competes with it in metabolism.
Antioxidant	An agent that prevents or inhibits oxidation of a substance by combing with oxygen.
Apoenzyme	The inactive protein part of an enzyme that remains after the cofactor is removed.
Avidin	A glycoprotein found in raw egg whites that binds biotin in the intestinal tract and inhibits the absorption of biotin.
Basal metabolic rate (BMR)	The rate at which the body uses oxygen when it is at rest and food has not been ingested for 12 hours.
Basic amino acids	Amino acids whose side chains have positively charged amino groups.
β-carotene	A carotinoid that is a precursor of Vitamin A found in plant foods.
β-oxidation	The enzymatic process that occurs in mitochondria whereby Fatty acids are oxidatively degraded at the second carbon atom from the carboxyl group.
β-Oxidation pathway	Fatty acid breakdown involves a repeating sequence of four reactions. Oxidation of the acyl CoA by FAD to form a trans-D^2-enoyl CoA; Hydration to form 3-hydroxyacyl CoA; Oxidation by NAD^+ to form 3-ketoacyl CoA;Thiolysis by a second CoA molecule to form acetyl CoA and an acyl CoA shortened by two carbon atoms. The $FADH_2$ and NADH produced feed directly into oxidative phosphorylation, while the acetyl CoA feeds into the citric acid cycle where further $FADH_2$ and NADH are produced. In animals the acetyl CoA produced in β–oxidation cannot be converted into pyruvate or oxaloacetate and cannot therefore be used to make glucose. However, in plants two additional enzymes allow acetyl CoA to be converted into oxaloacetate via the glyoxylate pathway.

Term	Explanation(s)
Bile pigment	A breakdown product of the heme portion of hemoglobin, myoglobin and cytochromes.
Bile salts	Derivatives of cholesterol that are synthesized in the liver and stored in the gallbladder.
Bilirubin	A bile pigment resulting from the breakdown of heme, the non-protein iron-containing portion of hemoglobin, myoglobin, and cytochromes.
Biliverdin	A product of the first step in the degradation of the heme portion of hemoglobin, myoglobin and cytochromes.
Black tongue	A disease seen in dogs that is an animal analog of pellagra, the niacin deficiency disease in humans.
Buffer	A substance or group of substances that resist a change in hydrogen-ion concentration of a solution.
Calmodulin	A calcium binding regulatory protein residing in the cytoplasm and affecting certain enzymes.
Calorie	A unit in which heat energy is measured.
Catabolism	Degradative reactions in metabolism.
Cellulose	A structural polysaccharide found primarily in plants and composed of glucose units bonded together by β–1,4 linkages.
Cephalin	A phospholipid, similar to lecithin, present in the brain of mammals.
Cerebroside	A lipid or fatty substance present in nerves and other tissues.
Chelation	A combination of metallic ions with certain heterocyclic ring structures so that the ion is held by chemical bonds from each of the participating rings.
Cholesterol	A high-molecular-weight cyclic alcohol contained in food of animal origin and synthesized in the body from Acetyl-CoA.
Chylomicron	A small lipid droplet composed mainly of dietary triacylglycerols, fat-soluble vitamins, small amounts of cholesterol and phospholipids, and a thin coating of protein.
Cofactor	A small, inorganic or organic substance that is required for the activity of an enzyme.
Collagen	The principal structural protein of bones, teeth, skin, cartilage, tendons, cornea, and blood vessels.

Term	Explanation(s)
Complete protein	A protein food that contains all the essential amino acids in relatively the same proportions, as humans require.
Cori cycle	The process by which lactate produced in skeletal muscles during contraction is recycled in the liver to glucose.
Degeneracy of the genetic code	One possibility is that degeneracy minimizes the deleterious effects of mutations. Degeneracy of the code may also be significant in permitting DNA base composition to vary over a wide range without altering the amino acid sequence of the proteins encoded by the DNA.
Diabetes mellitus	A disease in which the blood glucose concentration is unstable due to a relative or complete deficiency of insulin and a relative or great excess of glucagons.
Digestion	The enzymatic hydrolysis of food that occurs in the gastrointestinal tract. (deoxyribonucleic acid)
DNA	The molecule that carries, in the sequence of its bases, the genetic language of a species or an individual.
The principle of DNA cloning	Most foreign DNA fragments cannot self-replicate in a cell and must therefore be joined (ligated) to a vector (virus or plasmid DNA) that can replicate autonomously. Each vector typically will join with a single fragment of foreign DNA. If a complex mixture of DNA fragments is used a population of recombinant DNA molecules is produced. This is then introduced in to the host cells, each of which will typically contain only a single type of recombinant DNA. Identification of the cells that contain the DNA fragment of interest allows the purification of large amounts of that single recombinant DNA and hence the foreign DNA fragment.
The basis of DNA cloning	To clone into a plasmid vector, both the plasmid and the foreign DNA are cut with the same restriction enzyme and mixed together. The cohesive ends of each DNA reanneal and are legated together. The resulting recombinant DNA molecules are introduced into bacterial host cells. If the vector contains an antibiotic resistance gene(s) and the host cells are sensitive to these antibiotics, planting on nutrient agar containing the relevant antibiotic will allow only those cells that have been transfected and contain plasmid DNA to grow.

Term	Explanation(s)
DNA libraries	Genomic DNA libraries are made from the genomic DNA of an organism. A complete genomic DNA library contains all of the nuclear DNA sequences of that organism. A cDNA library is made using complementary DNA (cDNA) synthesized from mRNA reverse transcriptase. It contains only those sequences that are expressed as mRNA in the tissue or organism of origin.
Screening DNA libraries	Genomic and cDNA libraries can be screened by hybridization using a labeled DNA probe complementary to part of the desired gene. The probe may be an isolated DNA fragment (e.g., restriction fragment) or a synthetic oligonucleotide designed to encode part of the gene as deduced from a knowledge of the amino acid sequence of part of the encoded protein. In addition, expression cDNA libraries may be screened using a labeled antibody to the protein encoded by the desired gene or by using any other ligand that binds to that protein.
Dynamic state	A condition within a cell, tissue or organ in which a structure is constantly being produced and destroyed in such a way that there is no net gain or loss.
Electron acceptor	A member of an oxidation/reduction pair that can receive electrons from the electron donor; thus it is an oxidizing agent or oxidant. Oxygen is the ultimate acceptor in the respiratory chain.
Electron donor	A member of an oxidation/reduction pair that can donate electrons to an electron acceptor; thus it is an reducing agent or reductant. Hydrogen is a strong reducing agent whereas water is a weak reducing agent.
Energetic	The physical laws of energy and energy transformations that operate during every chemical reaction.
Energy yield from fatty acids	Complete degradation of palmitate (C16:0) in β-oxidation generates 35 ATP molecules from oxidation of the NADH and $FADH_2$ produced directly and 96 ATPs from the break down of the acetyl CoA molecules in the citric acid cycle. However two ATP equivalents are required to activate the palmitate to its acyl CoA derivative prior to oxidation. Thus the net yield is 129 ATPs.
Energy yield from citric acid cycle	For each turn of the cycle, 12ATP molecules are produced, one directly from the cycle and 11 from re-oxidation of the three NADH and one $FADH_2$ molecules produced by the cycle by oxidative phosphorylation.

Term	Explanation(s)
Enthalpy	The thermodynamic function of a system equivalent to the internal energy plus the product of the pressure and the volume.
Entropy	The randomness or disorder of a system. A measure of the capacity of a system to undergo spontaneous change.
Enzyme	A highly specialized protein molecule that serves as a catalyst for a specific chemical reaction and is not consumed or permanently altered by the reaction.
Enzyme inhibitor	A substance that reacts to modify the conformation of the active center or the substrate-binding site of an enzyme, slowing or preventing its catalytic action.
Ester	The product of a reaction of an acid with an alcohol in which water is removed.
Eukaryotes	Organisms whose cells contain a membrane bounded nucleus. With the exception of the bacteria and blue-green algae, all living organisms are eukaryotes.
Fatty acid synthesis	Fatty acid synthesis involves the condensation of two-carbon units, in the form of acetyl CoA, to form long hydrocarbon chains in a series of reactions. These reactions are carried out on the fatty acid synthase complex using NADPH as reductant. The fatty acids are covalently linked to acyl carrier protein (ACP) during their synthesis.
Role of fatty acids	They are components of membranes (glycerophospholipids and sphingolipids). Several proteins are covalently modified by fatty acids. They act as energy stores (triacylglycerols) and fuel molecules. Fatty acid derivatives serve as hormones and intracellular second messengers.
Favism	A hereditary condition common to persons native to the Mediterranean area resulting in sensitivity to a species of beans, *Vicia faba*.
Fiber	Polysaccharides for which humans do not have digestive enzymes; thus fiber contributes no calories to the human diet.
Fibrin	A protein synthesized from fibrinogen by the action of thrombin and required for blood clotting.

Term	Explanation(s)
Firinogen	A blood protein used to synthesized fibrin, a protein necessary for blood clotting.
Five classes of immunoglobulin	Human immunoglobulins exist as Ig A, Ig D, Ig E, Ig G and Ig M classes which contain α, δ, ε, γ, and M heavy chains, respectively. Ig M is a pentamer that binds to invading microorganisms and activates complement killing of the cells and phagocytosis. Ig G is the main antibody found in the blood after antigen stimulation and also has the ability to cross the placenta. Ig A mainly functions in body secretions. Ig E provides immunity against some parasites but is also responsible for the clinical symptoms of allergic reactions. The role of Ig D is unknown. All antibody molecules contain either Kappa (K) or Lambda (λ) light chains.
Free energy	The energy that is available to perform work as a biochemical system precedes towards equilibrium.
Function of cholesterol	Cholesterol is a component of cell membranes and is the precursor of steroid hormones and the bile salts.
Galactosemia	A metabolic inability, inherited as a recessive trait, to convert galactose to glucose because of an absence of galactose 1-phosphate uridyl transferase.
Glucagon	A polypeptide hormone secreted by the cells in the pancreas. Glucagon responds to low levels of blood glucose by activating cyclic AMP in the liver, thus stimulating gluconeogenesis and glycogenolysis.
Gluconeogenesis	The synthesis of glucose from substances such as lactate, some amino acids, and glycerol. The gluconeogenic pathway converts pyruvate to glucose.
Glycogenesis	The synthesis of glycogen. Glucose produced from the digestion and metabolism of carbohydrate and protein foods that are eaten in excess of need may be stored in glycogen molecules in the liver and muscles.
Glycogenolysis	The chemical process by which glucose is freed from glycogen. Glucose is a vital source of energy, especially for neutral tissues, and the body has evolved an exquisite method for its storage as glycogen as well as a smooth-running process for reclaiming it from glycogen.

Term	Explanation(s)
Glycolysis	A group of chemical reactions responsible for converting glucose to lactate and ATP without the consumption of oxygen, an anaerobic path. OR Glycolysis is a set of reactions that take place in the cytoplasm of prokaryotes and eukaryotes. The roles of glycolysis are to produce energy (both directly and by supplying substrate for the citric acid cycle and oxidative phosporylation) and to produce intermediates for biosynthetic pathways.
Half-life	The time required for half of a substance to disappear from a system.
Heme	The portion of hemoglobin, myglobin, and cytochromes that is responsible for their ability to carry and release oxygen and electrons.
Hemochromatosis	A rare disease of iron metabolism in which iron accumulations in body tissue. The liver becomes enlarged, the skin takes on a bronze hue, diabetes mellitus may develop, and cardiac failure is common.
Hemolysis	Rupture of red blood cells, resulting in anemia.
Henderson-Hasselbalch equation	An equation relating the pH, the pK, and the ratio of the concentrations of a weak base to that of a weak acid.
High density lipoprotein (HDL)	One of the lipoproteins in which lipids are carried in the watery fluids of the body.
High energy compounds	A substance whose hydrolysis results in the release of a large amount of energy.
Histidinemia	An accumulation of histidine in the blood and other tissues, resulting from the absence of histidase.
Holoenzyme	The complete, active enzyme. The protein parts, called the apoenzyme, plus the catalytic part, called the cofactor or coenzyme, make up the holoenzyme, which has biologic activity.
Homeostasis	A state of physiological equilibrium produced by a balance of functions and of chemical composition within an organism.
Homocystinuria	An inherited disease characterized by a high level of homocysteine excreted in the urine.

Term	Explanation(s)
Hormone	A chemical substance synthesized in one organ or gland that acts as a messenger to stimulate or inhibit the reactions in another organ or tissue. Hormones may be steroids, proteins or protein derivatives.
Hydrogenation	The process of adding hydrogen atoms to a substance to alter its physical or chemical characteristics.
Hydrolysis	The process by which a molecule is broken apart with the addition of water.
Hydrophilic	A descriptive term indicating that a molecule is polar (has regions of opposing charges) and associates with water molecules.
Hydrophobic	A descriptive term indicating that a molecule is nonpolar and is repelled by water molecules.
Hyperkalemia	A serum potassium level above 6 mEq/L. A level of 7 mEq/L is considered an emergency situation.
Hyperuricemia	An increase in the serum level of uric acid.
Hypokalemia	A serum potassium level below 3.5 mEq/L.
Immunoprotein	A protein, usually found in the gamma globulin fraction of blood plasma, that develops in response to an antigen and reacts with the antigen to cause its destruction.
Inositol	An alcohol that is a part of a phosphoglyceride in cell membrane structures.
Insulin	A hormone, secreted by the beta cells of the islets of Langerhans in the pancreas, that enhances the uptake of glucose by the peripheral tissues and thus maintains the blood glucose level within normal limits.
Intrinsic factor	A protein secreted by the gastric cells and required for the absorption of Vitamin B_{12}.
Isoelectric point	The pH of the solution at which a protein will posses an equal number of positively and negatively charged groups, i.e. the protein posses on net charge.
Isoprene	A five carbon unit important in the synthesis of many biochemicals known for their fragrance, such as bay leaves or menthol, and other molecules some of which lend colour to tomatoes and carrots.

Term	Explanation(s)
Jaundice	A yellow colour in the skin that is evidence of an accumulation of bilirubin, a bile pigment produced in the spleen during the breakdown of the heme portion of hemoglobin, myoglobin, and cytochromes.
Ketone bodies	When in excess, acetyl CoA produced from the β- oxidation of fatty acids is converted into acetate and D-3-hydroxybutarate. Together with acetone, these compounds are collectively termed ketone bodies. Acetoacetate and D-3- hydroxybutarate are produced in the liver and provide an alternative supply of fuel for the brain under starvation conditions or in diabetes, e.g., Acetoacetate, β-hydroxybutyrate and acetone.
Ketonemia	A high level of ketone bodies in the blood.
Ketonuria	A high level of ketone bodies in the urine.
Ketosis	Metabolic acidosis caused by a rise in the plasma level of the acids, acetoacetate, β-hydroxybutyrate and acetone.
Lecithin	The travel name of a phosphoglyceride whose correct name is phosphatidylcholine.
Lipogenesis	The synthesis of lipids.
Lipolysis	The hydrolysis of lipids by enzymes termed lipases.
Lipoproteins	Conjugated proteins consisting of simple proteins combined with lipid components, the latter including cholesterol, phospholipids or triacylglycerols. (Lipoproteins and their density: Chylomicrons <0.960, VLDL, 0.960 – 1.006, LDL, 1.006 – 1.059, HDL, 1.059 – 1.210, VHDL, 1.210 g/cm^3).
Melanin	The pigment of the skin and hair. It is derived from tyrosine through the action of the enzyme tryosinase to produce DOPA (3,4-dihydroxyphenylalanine).
Metabolism	The sum of all the biochemical changes that take place in a living organism (anabolism and catabolism).
Metabolite	Any intermediate compound produced during the catabolism of a biological substance.
Micelle	A very fine colloidal dispersion of polar lipids usually as a parallel array within a lipid phase, which fails to form a true solution of the molecules.

Term	Explanation(s)
Mutation	Chemical modification of a gene such that one or more of the bases in the DNA is deleted or altered or a new base is inserted, thus changing the base sequence.
Myoglobin	A heme protein that is abundant in muscles.
Nitrogen	The unique element in amino acids, purines, pyrimidines, and other nitrogenous biomolecules, the major component of the atmosphere, and the element on which the human food supply is most dependent.
Nitrogen balance	The nutritional state of an individual in relation to his or her protein metabolism; it is a measure of the difference between ingested and excreted nitrogen.
Osteoblasts	Cells responsible for forming new bone tissue.
Osteoclasts	Cells responsible for bone destruction by resorbing the calcium from bone.
Oxidase	A class of enzyme that is active in oxidation/reduction reactions, which use oxygen as an electron acceptor.
Pantothenic acid	A vitamin that play important biochemical role as part of the structure of coenzyme A.
PCR application	PCR has made a huge impact in molecular biology, with many applications in areas such as cloning, sequencing, the creation of specific mutations, medical diagnosis and forensic medicine.
Pellagra	A niacin deficiency disease.
pH	A numerical representation of the hydrogen ion concentration of a fluid that shows the acidity or alkalinity of the fluid.
Phosphoenol-pyruvate (PEP)	A high energy phosphate compounds that is an intermediate in both glycolysis and gluconeogenesis. Phosphoenolpyruvate has a much larger standard free energy of hydrolysis than ATP.
Phosphorylation	The process whereby a phosphate group is attached to a substrate for example when fructose 1-phosphate becomes fructose 1-6, diphosphate during glycolysis.
K'	A constant that is the pH at which the protonated and unprotonated components are equal. Stated in other terms pK' is the pH at which an acid is one-half dissociated. The pK' of each acid is unique.

Term	Explanation(s)
Polar	A substance having one region more negatively charged than another region.
Principles of PCR	The polymerase chain reaction allows an extremely large number of copies to be synthesized of any given DNA sequence provided that two oligonucleotide primers are available that hybridize to the flanking sequences on the complementary DNA strands. The reaction requires the target DNA, the two primers, all four deoxyribonucleotide triphosphates and a thermostable DNA polymerase such as Taq DNA polymerase. A PCR cycle consists of three steps, denaturation, primer annealing and elongation. This cycle is repeated for a set number of times depending on the degree of amplification required.
Prokaryotens	Simple cells having only a singe membrane.
Prosthetic group	A non-protein component attached to a protein that is generally necessary for the proteins biological activity.
Pyruvate	A key intermediate in the extraction of energy from glucose, some amino acids and glycerol.
Ribosome RNA	A highly organized assembly of RNA and protein molecules present in the cytosol.
Ribonucleic acid	Single strand molecules that are complementary copies of a segment of DNA. Some RNAs are in the information carrying business and some are in the protein building business.
Role of citric acid cycle	The main role of the citric acid cycle is the oxidation of pyruvate (formed during the glycolytic breakdown of glucose) to CO_2 and H_2O with the concomitant production of energy. It also has a role in producing precursors for biosynthetic pathways.
Saturated fatty acids	Fatty acids that contain only single carbon-carbon bonds.
Scurvy	A disease resulting from a deficiency of vitamin C.
Serum	The liquid portion of coagulated blood from which all cells and fibrinogen have been removed.
Sickle-cell-anemia	An inherited disease caused by an alteration in the beta chains of hemoglobin that results in a decreased ability of red blood cells to carry oxygen.

Term	*Explanation(s)*
Sodium pump **(Na^+ -K^+ pump)**	The energy requiring process by which a high concentration of potassium ions and low concentration of sodium ions are maintained inside nearly all animal cells.
TCA cycle	A series of catabolic reactions taking place in the mitochondrial matrix.
Urea cycle	A metabolic cycle taking place in the liver that prepares toxic ammonia for safe travel through the blood and then excretion by the kidney.
Vitamins	Organic substances needed by the body in tiny amounts, the dietary absence of which can cause specific metabolic defects. These substances may in some instances be synthesized by humans but may not be synthesized in sufficient quantity to support normal health.
Wilson's disease	A hereditary syndrome transmitted as a recessive trait in which liver proteins cause increased binding of copper.
Zymogens	An inactive enzyme that becomes active only in the presence of its substrate.

5

GENERAL INFORMATION

Most of the molecules in living systems contain only six different atoms: carbon, hydrogen, oxygen, nitrogen, phosphorus and sulphur. The outer electron shell of each atom has a characteristic number of electrons.

- When energy is released in any chemical reaction, LE is negative (-LE).
- When energy is consumed in any chemical reaction then the LE is positive (+LE).
- Types of bonds formed in various chemical reactions:
    1. Covalent bon (single bond),
    2. Double bond,
    3. Sigma bond,
    4. Hydrogen bond,
    5. Ionic bond.
- The power of an atom in a molecule to attract electrons to itself is called electron negativity.
- A molecule that incorporates separated positive and negative charges is called a dipole, e.g., water.
- Pure aqueous solution $[H^+] = [OH^-] = 10^{-7}$ M.
- PH = Log $[H^+]$ = $-\log 1/ [H^+]$, Where p = $-$ve log, H = $[H^+]$
- Any molecule or ion that can release a hydrogen ion is called an acid.
- Any molecule or ion that combine with a hydrogen ion is called a base.
- A dipolar ($-$ve or +ve) ion is called zwitterions.
- Molecules that bind to enzymes and increase or decrease their activities are said to be effectors of enzyme activity.
- Activators are positive effectors and inhibitors are negative effectors. The sites at which effectors binds are called regulatory or allosteric sites.
- The native state of DNA is a double helix of two antiparallel chains that have complementary sequences of nucleotides.
- RNA differs from DNA in its chemical structure and its three-dimensional folding.

- Fatty acids with no double bonds are termed saturated; those with at least one double bond are termed as unsaturated.

- A triacylglycerol consists of three fatty acid molecules and one molecule of glycerol.

6

SHORT EXPLANATIONS/REASONING

NITROGEN FIXING ORGANISMS

1. Free-living nitrogen-fixing organisms are given below:

Sr.No.	Habit when diazotrophic	Genus or type	Examples of species
1.	Strict anaerobes Archaebacteria	Methanosarcina	M. barkeri
		Methanococcus	M. thermolithotropicus
	Eubacteria	Bacillus	B. polymyxa, B. macerans
		Clostridium	C. pasteurianum, C. butyricum
		Desulfotomaculum	D. ruminis, D. orientis
		Desulfovibrio	D. desulfuricans, D. Vulgaris, D. gigas
2.	Facultative anaerobics	Klebsiella	K. pneumoniae, K. aerogenes
		Enterobacter	E. aerogenes, E. cloacae
		Escherichia	E. coli*
3.	Micro-aerobes	Aquaspirillum	A. perigrenum, A. fasciculus
		Arthrobacter	A. fluorescens
		Azospirillum	A. lipoferum, A. brasilense
4.	Aerobes	Azobacter	A. beijerinckii, A. chroococcum, A. vinelandii
		Beijerinckia	B. derxii, B. indica, B. mobilis
		Derxia	D. gummosa
5.	Photosynthetic bacteria	Rhodospeudomonas	R. palustis, R. capsulata, R. viridis
		Rhodospirillum	R. rubrum, R. tenue, R. fulvum
		Chromatium	C. vinosum, C. minus, C. weissei
6.	Cyanobacteria (aerobic)	Anabaena, Cylinfrosperma, Nostoc, Catothrix	-

* *Escherichia coli*, by genetic transfer of genes from *Klebsiella pneumoniae*.

2. Symbiotic Systmes

1. Rhizobium - Legume associations, Legumes + Rhizobium (leguminosarum: Biovar-trifolii, Phaseoli, Viceae, Meliloti, Loti)

2. Bradyrhizobium - Legume associations, Legumes + Bradyrhizobium (Japonicum sp.).

3. Bradyrhizobium – Non-legume associations, Parasponia + B. parasponia.

4. Framkia (actinomycete) – Non-legume associations, Nonlegumes.

5. Azotobacter paspali, Azospirillum-tropical grasses associations.

6. Cyanobacterial associations:
    (a) With angiosperms
    (b) With gymnosperms
    (c) With pteridophytes
    (d) With bryophytes
    (e) Lichens

Mechanism of Nitrogen Fertilizer Synthesis

The technology for manufacturing ammonia was developed by German scientists shortly before World War I. The raw materials for the process are nitrogen from the atmosphere and hydrogen, which can be obtained from many sources. In the United States, more than 95% of ammonia is made using hydrogen from natural gas, which is largely methane in a series of reactions that take place at high temperatures and pressures in the presence of catalysts. The methane is broken down into hydrogen in the following reaction:

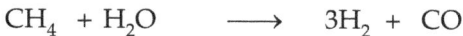

$$CH_4 + H_2O \longrightarrow 3H_2 + CO$$

The hydrogen and nitrogen from the atmosphere react, again at high temperatures and pressures in the presence of catalysts to produce ammonia.

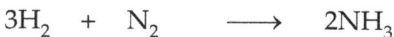

$$3H_2 + N_2 \longrightarrow 2NH_3$$

The ammonia can be used directly as a fertilizer or it can be reacted with a number of acids to produce various forms of fertilizers, including;

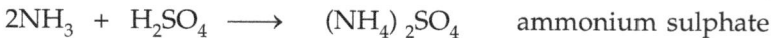

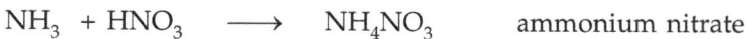

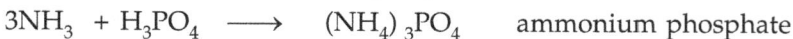

$$2NH_3 + H_2SO_4 \longrightarrow (NH_4)_2SO_4 \quad \text{ammonium sulphate}$$
$$NH_3 + HNO_3 \longrightarrow NH_4NO_3 \quad \text{ammonium nitrate}$$
$$3NH_3 + H_3PO_4 \longrightarrow (NH_4)_3PO_4 \quad \text{ammonium phosphate}$$

At high temperature and pressure, urea fertilizer can be produced by reacting ammonia and carbon dioxide in a two-step process.

First step:

$$2NH_3 + CO_2 \longrightarrow NH_2COONH_4 \quad \text{ammonium carbamate}$$

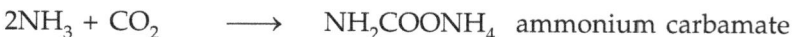

Second step: The product is then dehydrated to form urea.

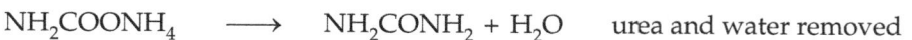

$$NH_2COONH_4 \longrightarrow NH_2CONH_2 + H_2O \quad \text{urea and water removed}$$

What are the principal differences between prokaryotic and eukarytic cells?

The detail differences are given below:

Characteristic	Eukaryotes		Prokaryotes
	Higher plant	Animal	
Number of chromosomes	> 1	> 1	1
Nucleoplasm bounded by a membrane	+	+	-
Histones	+	+	-
Nucleolus	+	+	-
Nuclear division by mitosis Organelles	+	+	-
Endoplastic reticulum	+	+	-
Golgi vesicles	+	+	-
Mitochondria	+	+	-
Chloroplasts	+	+	-
Peroxisomes	+	+	-
Vacuoles	+	-	-
Cell wall containing Cellulose	+	-	-
Peptidoglycan	-	-	+

+ Presence, - Absence

Chromosome Numbers of Various Species

The chromosome numbers of various species such as animals, haploid plants and fungi, diploid plants and fungi are given below:

Common name	Diploid/ Chromosome number	Common name	Diploid/ Chromosome number
Animals		Guinea pig	64
Alligator	32	Horse	64
Cat	38	Housefly	12
Cattle	60	House mouse	40
Chicken	78	Human	46
Crap	104	Mold (fungus)	8
Dog	78	Nematode	11M, 12F
Flatworm	16	Penicillin mold	4
Freshwater hydra	32	Pink bread mold	7
Frog	26	Rabbit	44
Fruit fly	8	Rat	42
Golden hamster	44	Rhesus monkey	42
Green algae	16	Silkworm	56

Common name	Diploid/ Chromosome number	Common name	Diploid/ Chromosome number
Slime mold	7	Coconut	32
Diploid plant and fungi	**Diploid number**	Coffee	22
		Coriander	22
Agathi	24	Corn	20
Almond	16	Cow pea	22
Amaranthus	32	Crambe	90
Aonla	28	Cucumber	14
Apple	34	Custard apple	14
Apricot	16	Date palm	36
Areca nut	32	Dolichos bean	22
Asparagus	20	Drum stick	28
Avocado	24	Elephant foot yam	26
Bael	18	Endive	18
Banana	22,33,44	Fenugreek	16
Barley	14	Fig	56
Barnyard	36, 54	Finger millet	40
Beet root	18	Foxtail millet	18
Ber	48 (4x)	French bean	22
Bitter gourd	22	Garden onion	16
Bottle gourd	22	Garden pea	14
Brinjal	24	Garlic	16
Broad bean	12	Gherkin	24
Brussel's sprout	18	Globe artichoke	34
Bullock's heart	14	Grape	38
Cabbage	18	Grape fruit	18
Carambola	24	Greater yam	40
Carrot	18	Green algae	20+
Cashew	42	Guava	22
Cassava	36	Ivy gourd	24
Cauliflower	18	Jack fruit	56
Celery	22	Jamun	40
Chekurmanis	-	Jerusalem artichoke	102
Chicory	18	Jojoba	52
Chilli	24	Kagzi lime	18
Chines cabbage	20	Kale	18
Chinese potato	-	Karonda	22
Chive	16	Kidney bean	22
Chow-chow	28	Kiwi fruit	58
Cluster bean	14	Knol-Khol	18
Cocao	20	Kodo millet	36

Contd...

Common name	Diploid/ Chromosome number	Common name	Diploid/ Chromosome number
Leaf mustard	36	Pointed gourd	22
Leek	32	Pomegranate	18
Lemon	18	Poppy	22
Lesser yam	40		
Lettuce	18	Ridge gourd	26
Lima bean	-	Round melon	22
Litchi	30	Sapota	26
Little millet	36	Sawa	54
Long melon	24	Shallot	16
Loquat	34	Snake gourd	22
Macadamia nut	48	Snapdragon	16
Mandarin	18	Snapmelon	24
Mango	40	Sorghum	20
Mangosteen	24	Spinach	12
Musk melon	24	Spine gourd	28
Oil palm	32	Sponge gourd	26
Okra	130	Sprouting Broccoli	18
Onion	48	Straw berry	56
Palak	18	Summer squash	40
Palmyra	32	Sweet cherry	16
Papaya	18	Sweet corn	20
Passion fruit	18	Sweet orange	18
Peach	16	Sweet pepper	24
Pear	34	Sweet potato	90
Peas	14	Tamarind	24
Pecanut	36	Tannia	26
Persimmon	90	Taro	28
Phalsa	36	Tea	30
Pine	24	Teff	40
Pineapple	50	Tobacco	48
Pistachio nut	30	Tomato	24
Plum	16 (Japanese) 48 (European)	Turnip	20
		Walnut	32
Potato	48	Water melon	22
Proso millet	36	Wax gourd	24
Pumkin	40	White yam	40
Radish	18	Winged bean	18
Rice	24	Winter squash	40
		Wood apple	18
		Yeast	36+

CARBOHYDRATES

Carbohydrates are carbon compounds that contain hydrogen and oxygen in the ratio 2:1. Chemically carbohydrates are aldehyde or ketone derivatives of polyhydric alcohols; these are known as aldoses or ketoses. Hydrated carbons are also called carbohydrates.

Classification of Carbohydrates

A. Monosaccharides

Glyceraldehyde	Lyxoketose	Talose
Dihydroxyacetone	Ribulose	Atrose
Erythrose	Xylulose	Allose
Threose	Fructose	Glucoheptose
Xyloketose	Sorbose	Mannoheptose
Arabinose	Glucose	Sedoheptulose
Xylose	Mannose	Glucooctase
Ribose	Galactose	Mannooctase
Lyxose	Gulose	Mannononose
	Idose	Glucodecose

B. Disaccharides

I. Reducing sugars

Maltose α–1, 4 Glucose + Glucose

Lactose β–1, 4 Glucose + Galactose

Cellobiose β–1, 4 Glucose + Glucose

Gentiobiose β–1, 6 Glucose + Glucose

Melibiose α–1, 4 Glucose + Galactose

Isomaltose α–1, 6 Glucose + Glucose

II. Non-reducing sugars

Sucrose α–1, b-2 Glucose + Fructose

Trehalose α-1, b-2 Glucose + Glucose

C. Trisaccharides

    I. Reducing sugars

Mannotriose	Galactose + Galactose + Glucose
Robinose	Galactose + Rhamnose + Rhamnose
Rhamninose	Galactose + Rhamnose + Rhamnose

    II. Non-Reducing sugars

Raffinose	Fructose + Glucose + Galactose
Gentobiose	Fructose + Glucose + Glucose
Melezitose	Glucose + Fructose + Glucose

D. Oligosaccharides

Stachylose	Fructose + Glucose + Galactose + Galactose
Verbascose Galactose	Fructose + Glucose + Galactose + Galactose +
Ajugose	Fructose + Glucose + Galactose + Galactose + Galactose + Galactose

E. Polysaccharides

    I. Homopolysaccharides

        Starches

        Dextrins

        Glycogens

        Celluloses

        Inulin

        Chitin

        Dextrans

    II. Heteropolysaccharides

        Agar

        Mucilages

        Gumarabic

        Gumacacia

        Pectins

        Alginic acids

III. Mucopolysaccharides

      Hyaluronic acid

      Heparin

      Chondroitin sulfates

      Sialic acids

    Which saccharides present in honey?

    Following different saccharides are present in honey:

Maltose, Sucrose, Gentiobiose, Isokestose, Kojibiose, Maltulose, Erlose, Melezitose, Turanose, Nigerose, Panose, Isomaltotetrose, Isomaltose, α, β-trehalose, Maltotriose etc.

Relative sweetness of different sugars

Sugar	Relative sweetness
Sucrose	100
Fructose	170
Glucose	70
Galactose	32
Maltose	30
Lactose	16
Lactulose	55
Saccharin	40000 - 50000

Sweetness of polyols

Sugar polyol	Relative sweetness
Gucitol	50
Lactitol	40
Maltitol	68
Mannitol	40
Xylitol	90
Sorbitol	63
Galactitol	58

Different Sugar Alcohols Present in Higher Plants

- Pentitol: Ribitol

- Hexitols: Sorbitol, D-Mannitol, Dulcitol, Allitol, L-Iditol, Polygalitol, Styracitol, and Hamamalitol

- Heptitols: Volemitol, Perseitol
- Octitol: D-Erythro-D-galacto-octitol

Properties of Amylose and Amylopectin

Property	Amylose	Amylopectin
Molecular configuration	Essentially linear	Highly branched
Weight-average (mol. Wt.)	Ca. 10^6	Ca. 10^8
X-ray diffraction	Crystalline	Amorphous
Action of β-amylase and Z-enzyme	Complete hydrolysis	Residual dextrin of high mol.wt.
Complex formation with iodine and polar substances	Readily forms complexes	Very limited complexes formation
Stability in aqueous solution	Unstable, tends to retrograde	Stable

Starch Degrading Enzymes

Enzyme	Reaction catalyzed
α-amylase	Hydrolytic cleavage of α-1, 4 bonds in a glucan
β-amylase	Liberation of maltose from the non-reducing end of a glucan
α-glucosidase	Hydrolytic cleavage of α-1- 4, or α-1- 6, bonds in oligosaccharides
Debranching enzyme	Hydrolysis of α-1 – 6 bonds
D-enzyme	G donor + G acceptor ↔ G donor + acceptor-1, + Glucose
Glucosyl-glucan transferase	Transfer of glycosyl, maltosyl or maltotriosyl residues to glucose
Phosphorylase	Glucose 1 – P + α-glucan ↔ α-glucose 1 – P + Glucose
Maltose phosphorylase	Matose + Orthophosphate ↔ Glucose –1-P + glucose

Fiber

Dietary fiber includes all remnants of plant cells, which are resistant to digestion by the alimentary enzymes of humans.

Crude fiber (CF) = Cellulose

Acid detergent fiber (ADF) = Cellulose + Lignin

Neutral detergent fiber (NDF) = Cellulose + Lignin + Hemicelluloses

Total dietary fiber (TDF) = NDF + Pectin + Gum + Mucilage

Structural polysaccharides: Cellulose and noncellulosic polysaccharides

Structural nonpolysaccharides: Gums and mucilages

Plant cell wall	Cellulose
Structural	Polysaccharide
Hemicellulose	Non-carbohydrate polymer
Lignin	Plant non-structural substances and food additives pectin, gums, mucilages and modified polysaccharides.

- If there are four different atoms or functional groups singly bonded to a carbon atom in an organic molecule the carbon atom is said to be **asymmetric**. Since it can exist two isomeric forms called **stereoisomers**. The two different mirror images of a molecule, which are not super imposable are called **enantiomers**.

- A molecule, which has only one asymmetric carbon atom that two ring, forms (α and β) and these are known as **anomers**.

- When D (+)-glucose is dissolved in water, a specific rotation of + 113 degrees is obtained, but this slowly changes, so that at 24 h the value has becomes + 52.5 degrees. This phenomenon is known as **mutarotation**.

- Monochromatic light passes through a Nicol prism and emerges polarized in one plane. This polarized beam then passes through the sugar sample, which rotates the plane of the light. This phenomenon is known as polarization or specific rotation of particular sugar.

  Specific rotation $[\alpha]^t_\lambda = \alpha/1 \times c$

  Where: Path length (ψdm), concentration of solution (c, g/ml), Temperature (t, °C), Wave length (λ nm), l = 589 nm, t = 20°C

- **Epimers :** Two stereoisomerisms differing in configuration at one asymmetric center in a compound having two or more asymmetric centers.

- Same molecular formula but different arrangement in the space of a molecule is known as **isomerism**.

  Types of isomerism : 1. Structural isomerism and 2. Stereoisomerisms.

  Structural isomerism : 1. Chain isomerism, 2. Positional isomerism and 3. functional group isomerism.

  Stereoisomerism : 1. Optical isomerism, 2. Geometrical isomerism

- **The pasture effect :** When oxygen is admitted to an anaerobic suspension of cells utilizing glucose at a high rate, the rate of glucose consumption declined dramatically as the added oxygen is consumed. In addition the accumulation of lactate ceased. Louis Pasteur observed this effect in 1860 so it is known as Pasteur effect.

- **Crabtree effect :** The Crabtree effect appears to be due to increased competition of glycolytic processes for inorganic phosphate and possibly pyridine nucleotides leaving less for oxidative phosphorylation reactions.

Major Factors Influences Carbohydrate Tolerances

Carbohydrate starvation

Effect of exercise

Hyper insulinism

Diseases of the liver

Acute and chronic infections

Thiamine deficiency

Nervous disorders

Effect of anesthetics and other drugs

- Starch is storage homopolysaccharide mostly present in plants and it consists of amylose and amylopectin.
- The partial hydrolysis of starch by acids or α - and β - amylases produces small substances known as dextrins.
- The larger branched dextrins give a red colour with iodine and are called as **"erythro-dextrin"**.
- The aldehyde and primary alcohol groups of aldoses can be oxidized to the corresponding **aldonic** or **uronic acids** and further oxidation of these acids yields **Saccharic acid**.
- Both aldoses and ketoses may be reduced to the corresponding polyhydroxy alcohols.
- The sugar alcohols are well-crystallized compounds soluble in water and alcohol and they have a sweet taste.
- Enolization takes place due to the action of alkalis on sugars.
- When sugars react with phenyl hydrazine it forms osazone.
- The hydrolysis of sucrose and formation of the equimolar mixture of glucose and fructose is known as invert sugar.
- General tests for chemical properties of carbohydrates:
  - Molisch's test
  - The anthrone reaction
  - Benedict's test
  - Phloroglucinol-hydrochloric acid test
  - Naphtho resorcinol test
  - Benzidine test

- Barfoed's test
- Iodine test
- Osazone formation test
- Seliwanoff's test (Resorcinol hydrochloric acid test)

- Preparation of osazones
- Bial's test for pentoses
- Tests for sucrose

ATPs evolved during complete oxidation of glucose

Reaction sequence	ATP yield/Glucose
Glycolysis: Glucose to pyruvate (in the cytosol)	
Phosphorylation of glucose	-1
Phosphorylation of fructose 6-phosphate	-1
Dephosphorylation of 2 molecules of 1,3-DPG	+2
Dephosphorylation of 2 molecules of phosphoenol pyruvate 2 NADH are formed in the oxidation of 2 molecules of glyceraldehydes 3-phosphate	+2
Conversion of pyruvate to acetyl CoA (inside mitochondria) 2 NADH are formed	
Citric acid cycle (inside mitochondria) Formation of 2 molecules of guanosine triphosphate from 2 molecules of succinyl CoA	+2
6 NADH are formed in the oxidation of 2 molecules of isocitrate, α-ketoglutarate and malate	
$2FADH_2$ are formed in the oxidation of 2 molecules of succinate	
Oxidative phosphorylation (inside mitochondria)2NADH formed in the glycolysis; each yields 2ATP (not 3ATP each, because of the cost of the shuttle)	+4
2NADH formed in the oxidative decarboxylation of pyruvate; each yields 3ATP	+6
$2FADH_2$ formed in the citric acid cycle; each yields 2ATP	+4
6NADH formed in the citric acid cycle; each yields 3ATP	+18
Net	**+36**

The overall reaction is:

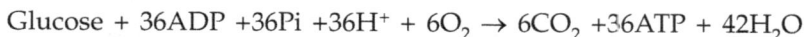

Glucose + 36ADP +36Pi +36H^+ + 6O_2 → 6CO_2 +36ATP + 42H_2O

The P:O ratio is 3 since 36 ATP are formed and 12 atoms of oxygen are consumed. The vast majority of the ATP, 32 out of 36 is generated by oxidative phosphorylation. The overall efficiency of ATP generation is high. The oxidation of glucose yields 686 Kcal under standard conditions;

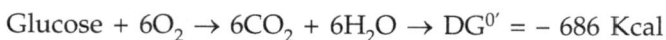

Glucose + 6O_2 → 6CO_2 + 6H_2O → $DG^{0'}$ = − 686 Kcal

The free energy stored in 36 ATP is 263 Kcal, since for hydrolysis of ATP is −7.3 Kcal. Hence, the thermodynamic efficiency of ATP formation from glucose is 263/686 or 38% under standard conditions.

Biochemical Functions of Carbohydrates

- Source of energy
- Conversion of solar energy in to chemical energy
- Central to metabolism
- Utilization of fats
- Sweetness of food
- Appetizing and flavouring
- Bulk of food
- Peristaltatic movement of stomach
- Movement of joints
- Structural support
- Storage of food material
- Transport between cells and organs
- Accumulation of fats
- Helps in pollination
- Helps in transamination
- Helps for fat burns
- Responsible for ketone body formation
- It exerts sparing effect of protein
- It acts as drugs
- It helps in protein synthesis
- Responsible for colour development to the products
- The ability to bind water and control water activity in foods is one of the most important properties of carbohydrates
- It helps in the sugar-flavourant formation
- Burnt carbohydrates gives colour to the food products
- It also acts as a lubricant at joints

Amino Acids and Proteins

Amino acids : Amino acids are organic compounds that contain amino and carboxyl group on the carbon atom and posses both acidic and basic properties.

Sr.No.	Group	Name	Abbreviation	Mol. Wt.
1.	Aliphatic	Glycine	Gly	75
		Alanine	Ala	89
		Valine	Val	117
		Leucine	Leu	131
		Isoleucine	Ile	131
2.	Hydroxylic	Serine	Ser	105
		Threonine	Thr	119
		Hydroxyproline	Hyp	131
3.	Sulphur	Cysteine	Cys	121
		Cystine	Cys-Cys	240
		Methionine	Met	149
4.	Acidic	Aspartic acid	Asp	133
		Glutamic acid	Glu	147
5.	Basic	Lysine	Lys	146
		Arginine	Arg	174
		Asparagine	Asn	132
		Glutamine	Gln	146
6.	Aromatic (Hetrocyclic)	Phenylalanine	Phe	165
		Tyrosine	Tyr	181
		Trptophan	Try	204
		Histidine	His	155
7.	Imino acid	Proline	Pro	115

Essential and Non-essential Amino Acids to the Human Being

Sr. No.	Essential amino acids	Non-essential amino acids
1.	Valine	Glycine
2.	Leucine	Alanine
3.	Isoleucine	Serine
4.	Phenylalanine	Aspartic acid
5.	Tyrosine	Glutamic acid
6.	Tryptophan	Proline
7.	Lysine	Cysteine
8.	Methionine	Threonine
9.	Arginine (For adults)	Asparagine
10.	Histidine (For children)	Glutamine
11.		Hydroxyproline
12.		Hydroxylysine

- Those amino acids are not synthesized in human body are known as the **essential amino acids**.

- While protein synthesis in the plant or in human body those amino acids excost first are known as **limiting amino acids**.

- The pH at which amino acid or protein posses zero net charge and no migration in an electric field is known as the **isoelectric point**.

- Amino acids exist in neutral solution as doubly charged ions known as **zwitterions** and not as unionized molecules.

- **Protein :** It is macromolecule composed of one or more polypeptide chains, each posing a characteristic amino acid sequence and specific molecular weight. Protein also defined as a polymer of amino acids.

Classification of Proteins

- Functional classification:
  - Storage proteins
  - Transport proteins
  - Catalytic proteins
  - Contractile or motile proteins
  - Structural proteins
  - Defense proteins
  - Immune proteins
  - Regulatory proteins
  - Other proteins
- According to shape:
  - Globular proteins
  - Fibrous proteins
- According to physical and chemical proteins
  - Simple proteins
  - Conjugated proteins
  - Derived proteins
- Combined proteins
  - Membrane proteins
  - Plasma proteins
  - Hormonal proteins

- • Enzyme proteins
- • Structural proteins
  - • Primary structural proteins
  - • Secondary structural proteins
    - • α-Helix proteins
    - • β-Plated sheet proteins
  - • Tertiary structural proteins
  - • Quaternary structural proteins

Simple proteins	Complex proteins
Protamines and Histones	Metal proteins
Albumins	Phosphoproteins
Globulins	Chromoproteins
Glutelins	Glucoproteins
Prolamins	Lipoproteins
Scleroprteins	Nucleoproteins
	Viruses

Seed proteins: Seed proteins from cereal grains are very heterogeneous and complex mixture of a large number of completely different types of molecules. All the individual molecular species of these proteins have not yet been isolated. Based on the solubility in various solvents, cereal proteins have been classified and separated into 4 major groups.

Albumin : Water-soluble

Globulin : Salt-soluble

Prolamine : Alcohol-soluble

Glutelin : Soluble in dilute alkali or acid

Albumin and globulin mainly function as enzymatic proteins, which carry out the metabolic processes in the grain, while prolamines, the major storage proteins are tissue-specific and are synthesized in the endosperm. They act as storage of nitrogen, carbon and generally sulphur and provide nutrition to the germinating embryo. Prolamines account for as much as 30-60% of the total grain protein in almost all cereals except rice. The essential amino acid composition of different protein fractions along with FAO reference protein indicates that albumin, globulin and glutelin are nutritionally more balanced while prolamines are extremely deficient in lysine and tryptophan. Since prolamines are the major proteins, they tend to lower the nutritional quality of cereal grains.

Protein Content and Prolamine Fraction of Cereal Grains

Cereal grain	Protein (% of dry weight)	Prolamine (% of total protein)
Wheat	10 –15	40 – 50 (Gliadin)
Maize	7 – 13	50 – 55 (Zein)
Barley	10 – 16	35 – 45 (Hordein)
Sorghum	9 – 13	60 (Kafirin)
Rice	8 – 10	1 – 5 (Oryzin)
Pearl millet	8 - 16	21 – 38 (Prolamine)

Classes of Secretary Protein in Vertebrates

Sr. No.	Type	Example	Sites of synthesis
1.	Serum proteins	Albumin	Liver (hepatocyte)
		Transferrin (Fe transporter)	Liver
		Immunoglobulins	Lymphocytes
		Lipoproteins	Liver
2.	Structural proteins	Collagen	Fibroblasts
		Fibronectin	Fibroblasts
3.	Peptide hormones	Insulin	Pancreatic β-islet cells
		Glucagons	Pancreatic α-islet cells
		Endorphins	Neurosecretory cells
		Enkephalins	Neurosecretory cells
		ACTH	Pituitary anterior lobe
4.	Digestive enzymes	Trypsin	Pancreatic acini
		Chymotrypsin	Pancreatic acini
		Amylase	Pancreatic acini, liver, Salivary glands
		Ribonuclease	Pancreatic acini
		Deoxyribonuclease	Pancreatic acini
5.	Milk proteins	Casein	Mammary gland
		Lactalbumin	Mammary gland
6.	Egg white proteins	Ovalbumin	Tubular gland cells of the avian oviduct
		Conalbumin	Tubular gland cells of the avian oviduct
		Lysozyme	Tubular gland cells of the avian oviduct

Present Sources of Energy (averaged over the earth's surface)

Sr. No.	Source	Energy in cal/(cm². Yr)
1.	Total radiation from sun	
2.	Ultraviolet light with wave length of	
	300 – 400 nm	3.4×10^3
	250 – 300 nm	5.6×10^2
	200 – 250 nm	4.1×10^1
	< 150 nm	1.7
3.	Electric discharges	4
4.	Shock waves	1.1
5.	Radioactivity (to 1.0 km depth)	8×10^{-1}
6.	Volcanoes	1.3×10^{-1}
7.	Cosmic rays	1.5×10^{-3}

Qualitative Tests for Amino Acids and Proteins

The list of tests for amino acids and proteins testing is given below:

- Solubility test
- The ninhydrin reaction test
- The xanthoproteic reaction test
- Millon's reaction test
- Glyoxylic reaction test
- Pauly's test
- Ehrlich's reagent test
- The nitroprusside test
- The sakaguchi reaction test
- The biuret test
- C – terminal amino test
- N – terminal amino test
- The Folin-Lowery method test

Protein quality parameters

- Total protein content
- True protein content
- *In-vitro* protein digestibility
- Net protein ratio

- True digestibility
- Protein efficiency ratio
- Biological value
- Calorific value
- Chemical score

Steps in protein synthesis

- Activation of amino acids
- Initiation of the polypeptide chain
- Elongation
- Termination
- Folding and processing

Multification factors while calculating protein content from different food and food products

Sr. No.	Food material	Multification factor
1.	Sorghum, Bajara/pearl millet, other millets and maize	6.25
2.	Rice	5.95
3.	Whole wheat	5.83
4.	Wheat bran	6.31
5.	Wheat flour (free from germ or bran)	5.70
6.	Bulgur wheat	5.83
7.	Rye	5.83
8.	Barley, Oats	5.83
9.	Groundnut (peanuts) and Brazil nuts	5.46
10.	Soybean	5.71
11.	Sesamum	5.30
12.	Sunflower	5.36
13.	Almonds	5.18
14.	Other nuts and oilseeds	5.30
15.	Casein and other milk proteins	6.38

Biochemical Functions of Proteins

- *Enzymes:* Metabolic catalysts, oxidation, synthesis etc.
- *Structural proteins:* Keratins-proteins of hair, hair, feathers, collagen-connective tissue fibers, muscle proteins, silk and chitin
- *Respiratory proteins:* Hemoglobin, cytochromes, myoglobin, and hemocyanin

- *Antibodies:* Proteins formed in response to antigens, protection against foreign proteins.

- *Hormones:* Regulatory of metabolism, e.g., insulin controls carbohydrate and fat metabolism.

- *Nucleoproteins:* Chromosomal proteins, control of hereditary transmission, ribosomal proteins, involved in protein synthesis.

- To replace the daily loss of body proteins.

- To provide amino acids for the formation of tissue during growth.

- To provide the amino acids necessary for the formation of enzymes, blood proteins, hormones are proteins in nature.

- To provide amino acids for the growth of fetus in pregnancy and for the production of milk during lactations.

- The structural proteins are fibrous proteins or chains proteins, keratin in skin, hair and nails, myosin in muscles.

- Proteins provide essential amino acids, which are not synthesized in the animal body.

- The blood and water balance of animal depends upon the osmotic pressure of plasma, serum albumin level.

Nitrogenous Compounds Occurring in Plants

- Ammonium
- Nitrate
- Proteins and their building blocks
- Enzymes of protein metabolism
- Fixation of elementary N
- Nitrification and denitrification
- Metabolism of proteins
- Amines and uridines
- Purines and pyrimidines
- Alkaloids

Proportion of Nucleic Acid in RNA

- Adenine   22.4
- Guanine   29.2

- Cytosine   27.6
- Uracil   20.8

Here the ratio A + U/G + C is 0.76, as composed with the ratio A + T/G + C + NC of 1.25 in DNA.

Nitrification and Denitrification

- **Nitrification**

The microbiological process, in which the ammonia content of soils is converted into nitrate. This conversion of primary importance for green plants, which can utilize nitrates N nutrients more readily than ammonium salts. Two bacterial types carry out nitrification in two consecutive reactions.

1. Nitrosomonas (nitrite bacterium)

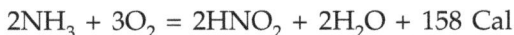

$$2NH_3 + 3O_2 = 2HNO_2 + 2H_2O + 158 \text{ Cal}$$

2. Nitrobacter (nitrate bacterium)

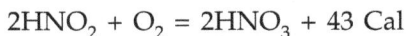

$$2HNO_2 + O_2 = 2HNO_3 + 43 \text{ Cal}$$

- **Denitrification**

1. $C_6 H_{12} O_6 + 4NO_3 = 6CO_2 + 6H_2O + 2N_2 + \text{about 420 Cal}$

2. Sulphur bacteria:

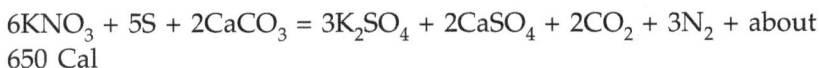

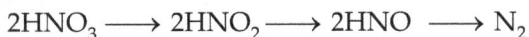

$$6KNO_3 + 5S + 2CaCO_3 = 3K_2SO_4 + 2CaSO_4 + 2CO_2 + 3N_2 + \text{about 650 Cal}$$

$$2HNO_3 \longrightarrow 2HNO_2 \longrightarrow 2HNO \longrightarrow N_2$$

LIPIDS

Lipids : lipids are naturally occurring compounds that are esters of long chain fatty acids.

What are the different classes of lipids and fatty acids?

1. Simple lipids   1. Saturated fatty acids

2. Compound or conjugated lipids   2. Unsaturated fatty acids

3. Derived lipids   3. Polyunsaturated fatty acids

What are the common saturated and unsaturated fatty acids found in lipids?

Common name	Symbol	Source
Butyric	4:0	Cow's milk
Caproic	6:0	Cow's milk
Caprylic	8:0	Milk, cocoa fat
Capric	10:0	Milk, palm oils
Lauric	12:0	Milk, palm oils
Myristic	14:0	Milk, coconut oil
Palmitic	16:0	All lipids and fats
Stearic	18:0	Milk, meats, pork, seed oils
Arachidic	20:0	Peanut oil
Behenic	22:0	Peanut oil, rapeseed oils
Lignoceric	24:0	Peanut oil, rapeseed oils
Myristoleic	14:1	Fish oils
Palmitoleic	16:1	Fish oils, milk
Oleic (ω9)	18:1	Major fatty acids
Cetoleic	22:1	Herring and other fish oils
Erucic (ω9)	22:1	Rapeseed oils
Ricinoleic	18:1	Castor bean, peanut oils
Linoleic (ω6)	18:2	
a-Linolenic (ω3)	18:3	Plant seed oils and fish oils
g-Linolenic (ω6)	18:3	
Arachidonic (ω6)	20:4	
Eicosapentaenoic (w3)	20:5	
Docosapentaenoic (w3)	22:5	Mostly fish oils
Docosahexaenoic (w3)	22.6	

Essential fatty acids are essential for dietary component for growth, reproduction eyesight and reduction in labour pains as well as menstrual sequence.

Which are the tests used for testing good quality of lipids?

- Saponification number
- Free fatty acids
- Iodine number
- Thiocyanogen number
- Peroxide value
- Acid number
- Polymorphism
- Absorption spectra

- Reichert-meissl number
- Polenske number
- Acetyl number
- Unsaponifiable matter
- Specific gravity
- Melting point
- Refractive index

Chemical Properties of Fats and Oils

- Hydrolysis
- Hydrogenation
- Halogenations
- Interesterification
- Acidolysis
- Rancidity
  - Oxidative rancidity
  - Hydrolytic rancidity
  - Ketonic rancidity
- Acetylation
- Oxidation
- Separation of fatty acids
- Ester formation

Waxes : Waxes commonly are defined chemically as the esters of higher fatty acids and of higher monohydroxy alcohols.

What are the classes of waxes?

- Lanolin or wool fat
- Bee's wax
- Carnauba wax
- Sperm oil

Steroids : Steroids have the parent nucleus of perhydrocyclopentano-phenanthrene, which consists of three six membered rings (A, B, and C) and a five member ring (D).

- Cholesterol
- Cholesterol
- Coprostanol

- Lanosterol
- Agnosterol
- Ergosterol
- Stigmasterol
- Sitosterol

Bile acids : Bile acids synthesize in pancreases and it helps in the digestion.

- Cholic acid
- Deoxycholic acid
- Lithocholic acid

How many ATPs are produced from oxidation of palmitic fatty acid?

The yield of ATP in the oxidation steps during oxidation of one molecule of palmitoyl-CoA to CO_2 and H_2O is given below:

Steps	NAD-linked steps	FAD-linked steps	ATP produced
Acyl-CoA dehydrogenase	-	7	14
3-Hydroxyacyl-CoA dehydrogenase	7	-	21
Isocitrate dehydrogenase	8	-	24
a-Ketoglutarate dehydrogenase	8	-	24
Succinyl-CoA synthetase	-	-	8
Succinate dehydrogenase	-	8	16
Malate dehydrogenase	8	-	24
Total ATP formed	31	15	131
Less 2ATP required for initial activation of palmitate (formation of CoA thiolester)			-2
		Net ATP	**129**

Biological Functions of Lipids

- Lipids act as a prime fuel reserve for metabolism. It is concentrated source of energy, yielding more than twice energy (2.25 times) supplied by carbohydrates or proteins per unit weight.
- Fats help to reduce the bulk of the diet as starchy food.
- Fats are essential for the absorption of fat-soluble vitamins *viz.*, A, D, E, K and especially carotenoids (vitamin A precursor) present in foods of vegetable origin.
- Fats improve the palatability of the diet.

- Some animal fat, e.g., fish liver oil, butter and ghee contain vitamin A and many vegetable foods contain vitamin E (wheat germ oil). Red palm oil is a good source of vitamin A.

- Fats are deposited in the adipose tissue. This deposit serves a reserve source of energy during starvation.

- Fat contains essential fatty acids *viz.*, linoleic, linolenic and arachidonic fatty acids, which are essential for maintaining the tissues in normal health.

- Fats are essential for the utilization of galactose present in glucose.

- Nearly 25-30% of the dry weight of brain consists of phospholipids. Lipids are essential constituents of nervous tissue.

- Fat is often deposited, largely subcutaneous in warm-blooded animals and serves as insulation against in unfavorable environment e.g., cold and physical injury.

- Waxes serves as a protective covering on the surface of an organism. The surface leaves, stems and fruits are rendered resistant to water, insects and bacteria by a wax coating.

- Fats are commercially important in the form of soaps, detergents grasses and the various oils of the paint industry.

- They are components of membrane (glycerophospholipids and sphingolipids).

  Several proteins are covalently modified by fatty acids.

- They act as energy store (triacylglycerols) and fuel molecules.

- Fatty acid derivatives serve as hormones and intracellular second messengers.

Ketone Bodies

When in excess acetyl CoA produced from the oxidation of fatty acid is converted into aceto acetate and D-3-hydroxybutyrate. Together with acetone these compounds are collectively termed ketone bodies. Aceto acetate and D-3-hydroxybutyrate are produced in the liver and provide an alternative supply of fuel for the brain under starvation conditions or in diabetes.

ENZYMES

Different Classes of Enzymes

- Oxidoreductase
- Transferases
- Lyases
- Hydrolases

- Isomerases
- Ligases

Factors Affecting Enzyme Activity

- Enzyme concentration
- Substrate concentration
- Temperature
- PH
- Concentration of any activators
- Concentration of any inhibitors

Properties of Enzymes

- All enzymes are protein in nature
- It has a catalytic property
- Heat labile
- Soluble in water, slightly soluble in acetone, alcohol and glycerol
- Having high molecular weight
- It reduce activation energy
- They form colloidal solution
- It accelerate the rate of reaction

Use of Enzymes

- It uses in digestive disturbances
- Used for healing of abnormal wounds
- Used for preparing protein hydrolates
- Enzymes used in fermentation
- Used in cheese, rennin making
- Used for clarification of fruit juices
- Used in wearing
- Used in leather industry
- Used in dry cleaning
- Used in preparing partially hydrolyzed products
- Used for recovering silver from photographic film
- Used in the production of different kinds of acids
- Used in analytical chemistry

Enzymes containing essential inorganic elements as cofactors

Inorganic element	Enzyme
Fe^{++} or Fe^{+++}	Cytochrome oxidase, catalase, peroxidase
Cu^{++}	Cytochrome oxidase, peroxidase
Zn^{++}	DNA polymerase, Carbonic anhydrase, Alcohol dehyrogenase
Mg^{++}	Hexokinase, Glucose-6-P, Pyruvate kinase
Mn^{++}	Arginase, Ribonucleotide reductase
K^+	Pyruvate kinase
Ni^{++}	Urease
Mo^+	Nitrate reductase, Dinitrogenase
Se	Glutathione peroxidase

Natural substrates of acid hydrolases located in lysosomes

Enzyme	Natural substrate
Phosphatases	
Acid phosphatase	Most phosphomonoesters
Acid phosphodiesterase	Oligonuclotides and other phosphodiesters
Nucleases	
Acid ribonuclease	RNA
Acid deoxyribonuclease	DNA
Polysaccharide and mucopoly saccharide hydrolyzing enzymes	
Galactosidase	Galactosides
Glucosidase	Glycogen
Mannosidase	Mannosides, glycoproteins
Glucuronidase	Polysaccharides and mucopolysaccharides
Lysozyme	Bacterial cell walls and mucopolysaccharides
Hyaluronidase	Hyaluronic acids; chondroitin sulphates
Arylsulfatase	Organic sulphates
Proteases	
Cathepsin	Proteins
Collagenase	Collagen
Peptidases	Peptides
Lipid-degrading enzymes	
Esterase	Fatty acyl esters
Phospholipase(s)	Phospholipids

Important oxidation-reduction reactions at pH 7.0 and 25°C?

Oxidant	Reductant	Number of electrons transferred
α-Ketoglutarate	Succinate + CO_2	2
Acetate	Acetaldehyde	2
Ferredoxin (oxidized)	Ferredoxin (reduced)	1
$2H^+$	H_2	2
NAD^+	$NADH + H^+$	2
$NADP^+$	$NADPH + H^+$	2
Glutathione (oxidized)	Glutathione (reduced)	2
Acetaldehyde	Ethanol	2
Pyruvate	Lactate	2
Fumarate	Succinate	2
Cytochrome β (+3)	Cytochrome β (+2)	1
Ubiquinone (oxidized)	Ubiquinone (reduced)	2
Cytochrome C (+3)	Cytochrome C (+2)	1
Fe^{+++}	Fe^{++}	1
½ O_2 + $2H^+$	H_2O	2

Pectic Enzymes Present in Plants

- Protopectinase
- Pectin-polygalacturonase
- Pectin-depolymerase
- Pectin-methylesterase

The degeneracy of the genetic code:

Number of synonymous codons	Amino acid	Total number of codons
6	Leu, Ser, Arg	18
4	Gly, Pro, Ala, Val, Thr	20
3	Ile	3
2	Phe, Tyr, Cys, His, Gln, Glu, Asn, Asp, Lys	18
1	Met, Trp	2
Total number of codons for amino acids		61
Number of codons for termination		3
Total number of codons in genetic code		64

Components of the mitochondrial electron transport chain

Enzyme complex	Mass (Daltons)	Prosthetic groups
NADH-CoQ reductase	85,000	FMN, FeS
Succinate-CoQ reductase	97,000	FAD, FeS
CoQH$_2$-Cytochrome C reductase	280,000	Heme b, c$_1$, FeS
Cytochrome C oxidase	2,00,000	Heme a$_1$, Heme a$_3$, Cu
Cytochrome C	13,000	Heme C

Enzymes take part in the metabolic pathways in cellular organelles

Organelle	Enzyme/Metabolic pathways
Cytoplasm	Amino trasnferases; peptidases, glycolysis, hexose mono-phosphate shunt; fatty acid synthesis, purine and pyrimidine catabolism
Mitochondria	Fatty acid oxidation; amino acid oxidation; Krebs cycle, urea synthesis, electron transport chain and oxidative phosphorylation
Nucleus	Biosynthesis of DNA and RNA
Endoplasmic reticulum (microsomes)	Protein biosynthesis, triacylglycerol and phospholipid synthesis; steroid synthesis and reduction; cytochrome P$_{450}$; esterase.
Lysosomes	Lysozyme, phosphoatases; phospholipases; hydrolases; proteases, lipases; nucleases
Golgi apparatus	Glucose-6 phosphatase; 5'-nucleotidase; glucosyl and galactosyl-transferases
Peroxisomes	Catalase; urate oxidase; D-amino acid oxidase; long chain fatty acid oxidation

VITAMINS, MINERALS AND HORMONES

- Vitamins are accessory food factors needed for the maintenance of good health and their absence from the diet leads to deficiency diseases.

- Hormones are chemical messengers produced by the endocrine glands and carried to the target organ they act to produce profound biochemical and physiological changes in the organism.

- These two groups of compounds are put together for convenience, as small quantities are needed to produce a large physiological or biochemical response. Apart from this vitamins and hormones are chemically different and are involved in a wide range of metabolic activities.

List of coenzymes, their precursors and deficiency disorder

Coenzyme	Precursor	Deficiency disease
Coenzyme A	Pantothenic acid	Dermatitis
FAD, FMN	Riboflavin (Vit. B_2)	Growth retardation
NAD, NADP	Niacin	Pellagra
Thiamine pyrophosphate	Thiamine (Vit. B_1)	Beriberi
Tetrahydrofolate	Folic acid	Anemia
Deoxyadenosyl cobalamin	Cobalamin (Vit. B_{12})	Pernicious anemia
Co-Substrate in the hydroxylation of proline in collagen	Vitamin C (ascorbic acid)	Scurvy
Pyridoxal phosphate	Pyridoxine (Vit. B_6)	Dermatitis

Typical ionic concentrations in invertebrates and vertebrates

Ion	Cell	Blood (mM)
Squid axon		
K^+	400 mM	20
Na^+	50 mM	440
Cl^-	40 – 150 mM	560
Ca^{++}	0.3 mM	10
X^{-+} (represents proteins)	300 – 400 mM	-
Mammalian cell		
K^+	139 mM	4
Na^+	12 mM	145
Cl^-	4 mM	116
HCO_3^-	12 mM	29
X^{-+} (represents proteins)	138 mM	9
Mg^{++}	0.8 mM	1.5
Ca^{++}	< 1 mM	1.8

Transport rate of sugars into the erythrocyte by facilitated diffusion

Sugar	Km (concentration required for a half-maximal rate of transport; mM)
D-Glucose	1.5
L-Glucose	> 300
D-Mannose	20
D-Galactose	30

Different biological functions of hormones?

Hormone	Functions
Growth hormone	Growth of bone and muscle
Thyroid stimulating	Synthesis and secretion of thyroxin
Follicle stimulating	Synthesis of estrogen
Leutizing	Synthesis of progesterone series
Interstitial cell stimulating	Synthesis of androgens
Prolactin	Stimulation of milk secretion ovarian function
Oxytocin	Contraction of smooth muscle milk ejection
Vasco pression	Water reabsorption contraction of smooth muscle
Melanocyte stimulating	Dilation leading to pigment dispersal
Pituitrin	Induces labour in child birth
Insulin	Carbohydrate metabolism, lower blood sugar
Glucogen	Increase blood sugar
Secretin	Secretion of salt and H_2O
Pancreozymin	Secretion of digestive enzymes
Enterogastrin	Stomach mobility
Gastrin	Acid secretion of stomach
Cholecystokinin	Contraction of gallbladder
Erythopoietin	Red blood cell formation
Relaxin	Relaxation of pelvic muscle
Parathyroid	Metabolism of calcium
Thyroxine	Metabolic rate, growth and development
Epiphrine	Break down of glycogen, increase of heart rate, blood pressure
Melatonin	Contraction of melanophores
Serotonin	Vasoconstriction
Aldosterone	Regulate salt and water balance
Testosterine	Testicular hormone
Progesterone	Precursor of corticoids, suppress estrus and ovulation
Estradiol	Induces estrus

Secondary compounds present in plants?

Group	Biosynthetic origin
Amino acids	Citric acid cycle, shikimic acid, others
Alkaloids	Amino acids, aromatic amino acids often with other pathways such as terpenoids, acetate
Alkanes, alkenes, aldehydes, alcohols, ketones, waxes	Acetyl-malonyl CoA (through fatty acids)

contd...

Group	Biosynthetic origin
Acetylenic compounds	Acetyl-malonyl CoA (through fatty acids)
Anthraquinoes	Polyketides or shikimic acid and mevalonic acid and others
Carbohydrates	Pentose cycle, photosynthesis
Cinnamic acids	Shikimic acid
Coumarins	Shikimic acid (through cinnamic acid)
Cyanogenic glucosides & lipids	Amino acids and carbohydrates or fatty acids
Fatty acids	Acetyl-malonyl CoA
Flavonoids	Aromatic amino acids and acetyl-malonyl CoA
Glucosinolates	Amino acids and carbohydrates
Phenyl propanoids	Cinnamic acids
Phenols (simple type)	Shikimic acid, acetylenic compounds, mevalonic acid, acetyl-malonyl CoA
Polyketides	Acetyl-malonyl CoA
Terpenes (steroids, carotenoids)	Acetyl-malonyl CoA (through mevalonic acid)

Radioisotopes commonly used in biochemical reactions

Isotope	Radiation	Half-life
^3H	β α	12.2 years
^{14}C	β	5700 years
^{22}Na	α	2.5 yeas
^{32}P	β	14.5 days
^{35}S	β	87 days
^{45}Ca	β	164 days
^{59}Fe	β, α	45 days
^{60}Co	α	5.25 years
^{125}I	α	60 days
^{131}I	β, α	8.1 days

Standard free energy produced during hydrolysis of some important compounds

Compound	ΔG (Cal/mol)
• High energy phosphates	
Phosphoenol pyruvate	-14.8
Carbamoyl phosphate	-12.3
Cyclic AMP	-12.0
1,3-Bisphospoglycerate	-11.8

Contd...

Compound	ΔG (Cal/mol)
Phosphocreatine	-10.3
Acetyl phosphate	-10.3
S-Adenosyl methionine	-10.0
Pyrophosphate	-8.0
Acetyl CoA	-7.7
ATP → ADP + Pi	-7.3
• Low-energy phosphates	
ADP → AMP + Pi	-6.6
Glucose 1-phosphate	-5.0
Fructose 6-phosphate	-3.8
Glucose 6-phosphate	-3.3
Glycerol 3-phosphate	-2.2

List of selected genes and their chromosome numbers

Genes	Chromosome number
Alkaline phosphatase	1
Apolipoprotein B	2
Transferrin	3
Alcohol dehyrogenase	4
HMG CoA reductase	5
Steriod 21-hydroxylase	6
Arginase	7
Carbonic anhydrase	8
Interferon	9
Parathyroid hormone	11
Glyceraldehyde 3-phosphate dehydrogenase	12
Adenosine deaminase	13
α_1-Antitrypsin	14
Cytochrome P_{450}	15
Hemoglobin α-chain	16
Growth hormone	17
Prealbumin	18
Creatine phosphokinase (M chain)	19
Adenosine deaminase	20
Superoxide dismutase	21
Immunoglobulin (λ chain)	22
Glucose 6-phosphate dehydrogenase	X
Steroid sulfate	Y

ALKALOIDS

Give the detail classification of alkaloids?

- Pyrrolidine, Piperidine and pyridine
- Piperidine alkaloid
    - γ-Coniceine
    - Interconversion of (+)-conine and γ-coniceine
    - Lobeline
- Pyridine
    - Ricinine
    - Nudiflorine
    - Nicotine
    - Nicotine synthetase complex
    - Nicccotine-Normicotine interconverion
    - Mimosine and related alkaloids
- Tropane alkaloids
- Amaryllidaceae alkaloids
- Quinolizidine (Lupine) alkaloids
- Quinoline alkaloids
- Isoquinoline alkaloids
- Morphine alkaloids
- Indole alkaloids
- Gramine
- Phalaristuberosa
- Ergot alkaloids
- Peptide ergot alkaloids
- Clavicipitic acid
- Fungal alkaloids
- Catharanthus alkaloids
- Steroidal alkaloids
    - Solanidine   Solasodine
      α-Solanine   α-Solamargine

β-Solanine	α-Solasonine
γ- Solanine	α-rhamnopyranosyl
α-Chaconine	β-D-glucopyranosyl
$β_1$-Chaconine	β-D-galactopyranosyl
$β_2$-Chaconine	
γ-Chaconine	

- Benzodiazepine alkaloids: Cyclopenine (Quinoline group)
- Purine alkaloids: Caffeine

• Hordenine	• Gramine
• Stachydrine	• Hyoscyamine
• Ephedrine	• Nicccotine
• Ricinine	• Mescaline
• N-Methylconiine	• Lycorine
• Colchicine	• Codeine
• Thebaine	• Morphine
• Pellotine	• Protopine
• Berberine	• Hydrastine

Major groups of isoflavonoids

• Isoflavone	⟶	Genistein
• Isoflavanone	⟶	Neotenone
• Rotenoid	⟶	Rotenone
• Pteroarpan	⟶	Glyceollin
• Isoflavan	⟶	Licoricidin
• Coumestan	⟶	Medicagol

Groups of phenolic acids?

- Cinnamic acid
- P-Cocumaric acid
- Caffeic acid
- Sinapic acid
- Ferulic acid

Cinnamic acids ($C_6 - C_3$ compounds)

- Cinnamyl alcohols
- Cinnamoyl amides
- Styrenes
- Benzoic acids
- Benzophenones
- Phenols
- Styrylpyrones
- Cinnamoyl esters
- Allyl phenols
- Acetophenones
- Flavonoids
- Xanthones
- Stibenes
- Coumarins

Benzoic acids ($C_6 - C_1$ compounds)

- Benzyl esters
- Benzyl alcohols
- Prenyl benzoic acids
- b-Glucogallin
- Benzoyl malic acid
- Benzaldehydes
- Phenols
- Ubiquinones
- Methyl salicylate
- Cocain

Phenylacetic acids ($C_6 - C_2$ compounds)

- Phenylpyruvic acid
- Homogentisic acid
- Toluhydro quinone

Typical alkaloids present in plants

- Ajmaicine
- Cytisine
- Berberine
- Codeine
- Aconite
- Emetine
- Solanine
- Atropine
- Galanthamine
- Colchicine
- Senecionine
- Strychnine
- Morphine
- Thebaine
- Quinine
- Skimmianine
- Chaconine
- Nicotine
- Tazettine

Different groups of quinines

- P-quinones
- O-quinones
- Benzoquinone
- Naphthoquinone
- Anthraquinone

Cyanogenic glucosides

- Linamarin
- (R)-Lotaustralin
- Linustatin
- Neolinustatin
- (S)-proacacipetalin
- Epiproacacipetalin
- (S)-heterodendrin
- (S)-cardiospermin
- Acacipetalin
- Vicianin
- Lucumin
- Dhurrin
- (R)-taxiphyllin
- (S)-cariospermin-p-hydroxybenzoate
- Amygdalin
- Deidaclin
- Gynocardin
- Proteacin
- Proteacin
- Prunasin
- Sambunigrin
- Taxiphyllin
- Triglochinin
- Zierin

Major and minor groups of flavonoids

Major groups

- Naringenin chalcone (chalcone) $\longrightarrow$ Naringenin (flavanone)
- Apigenin (flavone) $\longrightarrow$ Kaempferol (flavonol)
- Pelargonidin (anthocyanidin) $\longrightarrow$ Genistein (isoflavone)
  Minor groups:
- Bioflavonoid $\longrightarrow$ Amentoflavone
- C-Glycosyl flavonoid $\longrightarrow$ Vitexin

- Proanthocyanidin (condensed) $\longrightarrow$ Procyanidin
- Neoflavonoid $\longrightarrow$ Dalbergin

Plant toxins

The major classes of plant toxins are given below:

Class	Toxic activities	Organ distribution
A. Nitrogenous toxics		
Alkaloids (6000)	Many poisonous, hypnotic,. paralytic etc	Leaves, roots, fruits
Cyanogens (30)	Arrests respiration by blocking cytochrome system	Leaves, other tissues
Non-protein amino acids (300)	Neurotoxin, hypoglycemic	Mainly seeds
B. Non-nitrogenous toxins		
Iridoids (100)	Insecticidal, antimicrobial	Mainly leaves
Sesquiterpene lactones (600)	Allergenic cytotoxic	Leaf trichomes
Dierpenoids (600)	Co-carcinogenic, irritant	Mainly resins
Triterpenoids and steroids (3000)	Hemolytic cardio active	Leaves, roots, bulbs

Different pigmented compounds present in plants

- Anthocyanin pigments
- Yellow flavonoids
- Clourless flavonoids
- Betalain pigments
- Quinone pigments
- Carotenoid pigments

Plant anthocyanidins:

- Pelargonidin
- Peonidin
- Hirsutidin
- Capensinidin
- Apigeninidin

- Cyanidin
- Delphinidin
- Petunidin
- Malvidin
- Luteolinidin

Classification of plant anthocyanins

Simple

- Cyanidin 3-glucoside
- Cyanidin 3-rutinoside
- Cyanidin 3,5-diglucoside

Intermediate

- Cyanidin 3-Sinapyl-xylosylglucosyl galactoside (umbelliferae)
- Delphinidin 3-rhamnoside 5-glucoside (vicieae, leguminosae)

Complex

- Malvidin 3-(p-coumarylrutinoside) 5-glucoside (gesneriaceae)
- Cyanidin 3,7,3'- triglucoside (acylated with p-coumaric and ferulic) (commelinaceae)

Major classes of plant pigments

Sr.No.	Pigment class	Number of known structures
1.	Anthocyanins	300
2.	Yellow flavonoids	100
3.	Colourless flavonoids	600
4.	Betalains	50
5.	Quinonoids	300
6.	Carotenoids	400

Typical plant quinines

Benzoquinones

- Primin, glandular hairs, primula obconica
- Embelin, roots, myrsinaceae
- Dalbergione, Dalbergia heartwood

Naphthoquinones

- Plumbagin, plumbago root
- Juglone, Juglans

Anthraquinones

- Emodin
- Aloe-emodin
- Physcion
- Chrysophanol

Extended quinines

- Cyperaquinone
- Hypericin
- Hypericum

What are common carotenoids present in plants?

- β-Carotene
- α-Carotene
- γ-Carotene
- ε-Carotene
- Lycopene

- Zeaxanthin
- Rubixanthin
- Lutein
- Violaxanthin
- Crocin

Hidden metabolites present in plants and known to us

Class	Number of known structures
Fatty acids	150
Alkanes	50
Polyacetylenes	750
Storage sugars	50

High-energy bonds formed in the citric acid cycle

Reaction steps	Reaction	Number of high energy phosphate bonds formed
1.	Pyruvic acid + oxaloacetic acid + DPN = Citric acid + CO_2 + $DPNH_2$	0
2.	$DPNH_2$ +1/2 O_2 = DPN + H_2O	3
3.	Isocitric acid +TPN = a-ketoglutaric acid = + CO_2 + $TPNH_2$	0
4.	$TPNH_2$ + ½ O_2 = TPN + H_2O	3
5.	α-ketoglutaric acid + DPN = Succinic acid + CO_2 + $DPNH_2$	1
6.	$DPNH_2$ + ½ O_2 = DPN + H_2O	3
7.	Succinic acid + ½ O_2 = Fumarate + H_2O	2
8.	Malic acid + DPN = Oxaloacetic acid + $DPNH_2$	0
9.	$DPNH_2$ + ½ O_2 = DPN + H_2O	3
	Total	15
	Mean P/O	3

Colours occurrences by anthocyans in different plants

Anthocyan	Anthocyanidin	Glycoside	Occurrence	Colour
Callistephin	Pelargonidin	-3-monoglycoside	Callistephus	Red
Pelargonin	Pelargonidin	-3-5-diglycoside	Pelargonium Dahlia	Red
Monardaein	Pelargonidin	-3-5, diglycoside + 1 mole oxycinnamic acid + 2 moles malic acid	Red saliva	Red
Fragarin	Pelargonidin	-3-monogalactoside	Strawberry	Red
Paeonin	Cyanidin	-3-monomethyl ether	Peony	Red
Asterin	Cyanidin	-3-monglycoside	Aster	Violet red
Cyanin	Cyanidin	-3-5, diglycoside	Red rose, corn flower, leaves	Red or Blue
Idaein	Cyanidin	-3-galactoside	Cranberry	Red
Keracyanin	Cyanidin	-3-rhamnoglycoside	Black cherry, elderberry, blackberry	Bluish black
Prunicyanine	Cyanidin	glycorhamnoside	Plum	Blackish blue
Mecocyanine	Cyanidin	-3-gentiobioside	Poppy	Red
Petunin	Delphinidin	-3-monomethyl ether	Petunia	Bluish violet
Malvidin	Delphinidin	-3-5, dimethyl ether	Malva silvestris	Dark blue
Oenin	Delphinidin	-3-monoglycoside	Blue grape	Dark blue
Delphinin	Delphinidin	-Diglycoside	Larkspur	Blue
Violanin	Delphinidin	rhamnoglycoside	Pansy	Dark blue
Gentianin	Delphinidin	Glycoside + p-hydroxy cinnamic acid	Gentiana a caulis	Blue

Common aliphatic plant acids occurring most frequently

S. No.	Name of the acid	Structure
1.	Formic	$H.COOH$
2.	Acetic	$CH_3.COOH$
3.	Glycolic	$CH_2(OH).COOH$
4.	Glyoxylic	$CHO.COOH$
5.	Propionic	$CH_3.CH_2.COOH$
6.	Lactic	$CH_3.CHOH.COOH$
7.	Pyruvic	$CH_3CO.COOH$
8.	Glyceric	$CH_2OH.CHOH.COOH$
9.	n-Butric	$CH_3.CH_2.CH_2.COOH$
10.	Isovaleric	$CH_3.CH_3.CH.CH_2.COOH$

Contd...

S. No.	Name of the acid	Structure
11.	Oxalic	HOOC.COOH
12.	Succinic	$HOOC.CH_2.CH_2.COOH$
13.	Fumaric	HOOC.CH = CH.COOH
14.	Malic	$HOOC.CHOH.CH_2.COOH$
15.	Oxalacetic	$HOOC.CO.CH_2.COOH$
16.	Tartaric	HOOC.CHOH.CHOH.COOH
17.	Citric	$HOOC.CH_2.COH.CH_2.COOH$ COOH
18.	Isocitric	$HOOC.CH_2.CH.CHOH.COOH$ COOH
19.	Cis-Aconitic	$HOOC.CH_2.C = CH.COOH$ COOH
20.	Glyconic	$CH_2OH. (CHOH)_4.COOH$
21.	Glycuronic	HOOC.CHOH.CHOH.CHOH.CHOH.CHO
22.	Galacturonic	HOOC.CHOH.CHOH.CHOH.CHOH.CHO
23.	Ascorbic	CHOH.CHOH.CH.COH = COH.CO └——— O ———┘

7

DISTINGUISH BETWEEN/COMPARISON

Difference between prokaryotic and eukaryotic cells

Characteristic	Prokaryotic cell	Eukaryotic cell
Size	Small (generally 1-10 mm)	Large (generally 10-100 mm)
Cell membrane	Cell is enveloped by rigid cell wall	Cell is enveloped by a flexible plasma membrane
Sub-cellular organelles	Absent	Distinct organelles are found (e.g., Mitochondria, nucleus, lysosomes)
Nucleus	Not well defined; DNA is found as nucleoid, histones are absent	Nucleus is well defined, surrounded by a membrane; DNA is associated with histones
Energy metabolism	Mitochondria absent, enzymes of energy metabolism bound to membrane	Enzymes of energy metabolism are located in mitochondria
Cell division	Usually fission and no mitosis	Mitosis
Cytoplasm	Organelles and cytoskeleton absent	Contains organelles and cytoskeleton (a network of tubules and filaments)

Difference between oxidative phosphorylation and photophosphorylation

Sr. No.	Oxidative phosphorylation	Photophosphorylation
1.	In eucaryotics the oxidative phospjorylation occurs in mitochondria	In eucaryotics the photophosphorylation occurs in chloroplast
2.	Oxidative phosphorylation involves the reduction of O_2 to H_2O with electrons donated by $FADH_2$ or NADH	Photophosphorylation involves the oxidation of H_2O to O_{22} with $NADP^+$ as electron donor
3.	It occurs equally well in light or dark condition	Photophosphorylation absolutely dependent on light

Difference between reducing and non-reducing sugars

Sr. No.	Reducing sugars	Non-reducing sugars
1.	Reducing sugars have free OH group on anomeric carbon	No free OH group on anomeric carbon
2.	Exist as α- and β-isomers	No α- and β- isomers in same carbon
3.	Systematic name ends as -ose	Systematic name ends as -oside

Contd...

Sr. No.	Reducing sugars	Non-reducing sugars
4.	Many in number in the nature	Few in number in nature
5.	Gives reducing properties with metal ions such as copper, iron etc.	No reducing property with any metal ions.
6.	Example maltose, lactose, cellobiose, glucose, mannanose, galactose etc.	Example Sucrose, Trehalose, Reffinose, gentibiose etc.

Difference between light and dark reactions

Sr.No.	Light reaction	Dark reaction
1.	The light reactions which occur only when plants are illuminated	Dark reactions which can occur in the absence or presence of light
2.	In the light reactions chlorophyll and other pigments of the photosynthetic cells absorb light energy and conserve it in chemical form as the two energy rich products ATP and NADPH and O_2 evolved.	In dark reaction ATP and NADPH are used to produce CO_2 to form glucose and other organic products.
3.	O_2 occurs only in light reaction	CO_2 dose not require light
4.	Solar energy used for production of energy rich compounds	No need of sunlight energy
5.	It is dependant on sunlight	It is dependant on light reaction
6.	$2NADP^+ + 2H_2O + 2ADP + 2H_2PO_4 \xrightarrow{h\nu} 2NADPH_2 + O_2 + 2ATP$	$6CO_2 + 8ATP + 12 NADPH_2 + 12H_2O \xrightarrow{Reduced/Enzymes} C_6H_{12}O_6 + 18ADP + 18H_3PO_4 + 12NADP^+$
7.	That portion of the photosynthetic process in which light energy is converted into chemical energy	That portion of the photosynthetic process, which does not require light. Chemical energy in the form of ATP and reduced ferredoxin is produced from light energy in the light reaction and this chemical energy is used to carry on biosynthesis in the dark reaction.

Difference between C₃ plants and C₄ plants

Sr.No.	C_3 plants	C_4 plants
1.	First product is 3PGA	First product is oxalic acid, aspartic acid, malate
2.	CO_2 plants fixation in bundle sheath cells	CO_2 Fixation in mesophyl cells
3.	RuDP carboxylase enzyme take part in the reaction	PEP carboxylase enzyme take part in the reaction
4.	Low affinity for CO_2	High affinity to CO_2

Contd...

Sr.No.	C_3 plants	C_4 plants
5.	Photosynthesis efficiency is low	Photosynthesis efficiency is high
6.	Less energy required (i.e., 3ATP and 2NADPH)	High energy required (i.e., 5ATP and 2NADPH)
7.	Chlorophyll content is less (mostly a)	Higher chlorophyll content (mostly a and b)
8.	Temperate zone plants	Tropical zone plants
9.	Mesophyll cells are present in C_3 plants but do not make PEP	Photorespiration is very active in C_3 plants and it is practically absent in C_4 plants
10.	E.g., Millets, barley, wheat, pulses, mostly small/narrow leaves plants	E.g., Sugarcane, maize, sorghum, mostly broad leaves plants

8

BRAINSTORMING TERMINOLOGY

Term	Definition
Acetone; acetate	Acetone is a ketone; acetate is a carboxylic acid
Acetyl CoA; acyl CoA	Acetyl CoA is a specific compound containing acetate bound to coenzyme A; acyl CoA is a general term used to refer to any fatty acid (acyl group) bound to coenzyme A.
Amino; imino	Amino group ($-NH_2$) is found in majority of amino acids; imino group ($= NH$) is present in a few amino acids like proline and hydroxyproline
Anabolism; catabolism	Anabolism refers to the biosynthetic reactions involving the formation of complex molecules from simpler ones; catabolism is concerned with the degradation of complex molecules to simpler ones with a concomitant release of energy.
Anomers; epimers	Anomers refer to two stereoisomers of a sugar that differ in configuration around a single carbonyl atom; epimers are two stereoisomers that differ in configuration around one asymmetric carbon of a sugar possessing two or more asymmetric carbon atoms.
Apoenzyme; coenzyme	Apoenzyme is the protein part of the functional enzyme (holoenzyme); coenzyme is the non-protein organic part associated with enzyme activity.
Bile pigments; bile salts	Bile pigments (biliverdin, bilirubin) are the breakdown products of heme; bile salts are the sodium and potassium salts of bile acids (glycocholate, taurocholate) produced by cholesterol.
Biliverdin; bilirubin	Both are bile pigments. Biliverdin is produced from heme in the reticuloendothelial cells; bilirubin is formed by reduction of biliverdin.
Biotin; biocytin	Biotin is a B-complex vitamin; biocytin refers to the covalently bound biotin to enzymes (through e– amino group of lysine).

Term	Definition
B-Lymphocytes; T-lymphocytes	B-lymphocytes produce immunoglobins (antibodies) and are involved in humoral immunity; T-lymphocytes are responsible for cellular immunity.
Bisphosphate; diphosphate	Bisphosphate has two phosphates held separately e.g., 2, 3-BPG; diphosphate has two phosphate linked together e.g., ADP.
Calcitriol; calcitonin	Calcitriol (1, 25-DHCC) is the physiologically active form of vitamin D; calcitonin is a peptide hormone, synthesized by thyroid gland.
Calorimetry; colorimetry	Calorimetry deals with the measurement of heat production by organism; colorimetry is concerned with the measurement of colour compounds.
Carboxyl; carbonyl	These two are functional groups found in organic substance. Carboxyl group $-COOH$; carbonyl $-C = O$
Carnitine; creatine; creatinine	Carnitine transports activated fatty acids (acyl CoA) from cytosol to mitochondria; creatine is mostly found in the muscle as creatine phosphate, a high-energy compound; creatinine is the anhydride of creatine.
Choline; cholic acid	Choline is a trimethyl quaternary base and is a constituent of acetylcholine; cholic acid is an important bile acid.
Chyle; chyme	Chyle refers to lymph with milky appearance due to chylomicrons; chyme is the partially digested food in the stomach that passes to deodenum.
Cystein; cystine	Both are sulfur containing non-essential amino acids. Cysteine contains sulhydryl (-SH) group; cystine is formed by condensation of two cysteine residues and contains a disulfide (-S-S-) group.
Dextrins; dextrans	Both are polysaccharides composed of glucose. Dextrins are the breakdown products of starch; dextrans are gels produced by bacteria from glucose.
Diabetes mellitus; diabetes insipidus	Diabetes mellitus is primarily an important in glucose metabolism due to the deficiency of or inefficient insulin; diabetes insipidus is characterized by excretion of large volumes of urine (polyuria), caused by the deficiency of antidiuretic hormone (ADH).

Term	Definition
Endocytosis; exocytosis	Endocytosis is the intake of macromolecules by the cells; exocytosis refers to the release of macromolecules from the cells to the outside.
Epinephrine; norepinephrine	Both are catecholamines synthesized from tyrosine. Epinephrine is methylated while norepinephrine does not contain a methyl group.
Exons; introns	Exons are the DNA sequences coding for proteins; introns are the intervening DNA sequences that do not code for proteins.
GABA; PABA	γ-aminobutyric acid (GABA) is a neurotransmitter; p-aminobenzoic acid (PABA) is a vitamin.
Gene; genome	A gene refers to the DNA fragment of a chromosome that codes for a single polypeptide; all the genes of a cell or an organism are collectively known as genome.
Glu: Gla	Glu is the code for glutamic acid; Gla is the code for γ–carboxy glutamic acid.
Glucuronic acid; gluconic acid	Both are derived from glucose; oxidation of C_6 results in glucuronic acid while oxidation of C_1 yields gluconic acid. Glucuronic acid is produced in uronic acid pathway; gluconic acid is formed in hexose monophosphate shunt.
Glutaric acid; glutamic acid	Glutaric acid is a dicarboxylic acid; glutamic acid (a-amino glutamic acid) is an amino acid.
Glycogen; glycogenin	Glycogen is a storage form of carbohydrate (polysaccharide) in the animal body; glycogenin is a protein, which serves as a primer for the initiation of glycogen synthesis.
Glycoproteins; mucoproteins	Both are conjugated proteins containing carbohydrate as the prosthetic group. The term glycoprotein is used if the carbohydrate content is < 4%; mucoprotein contains > 4% carbohydrate.
Hydrophilic; hydrophobic	Hydrophilic refers to affinity to water; hydrophobic means hatred towards water.
Insulin; inulin	Insulin is a peptide hormone; inulin is a polysaccharide composed of fructose.
In vivo; in vitro	In vivo refers to within the cell or organism; in vitro means in the test tube.

Term	Definition
Isoniazide; iproniazide	Isoniazide is an antituberculosis drug; iproniazide is an antidepressant drug.
Lactam; lactim	These terms are used to represent tautomerism. Lactam indicates the existence of a molecule in keto form; lactim represents a molecule in enol form.
Linoleic acid; linolenic acid	Both are 18 carbon unsaturated fatty acids; Linoleic acid has two double bonds; linolenic acid has three double bonds.
Lipoproteins; lipotropic factors	Lipoproteins are molecular complexes composed of lipids and proteins; lipotropic factors are the substances (e.g., choline, betaine), the deficiency of which causes accumulation of fat in liver.
β-Lipoprotein; β-lipotropin	β-Lipoprotein refers to the low-density lipoproteins; β-lipotropin is a peptide hormone derived from proopiomelanocortin (POMC) peptide.
Lyases; ligases	Lyases are the enzymes that catalyse the addition or removal of water, ammonia, CO etc.; ligases catalyse the synthetic reactions where two molecules are joined together.
Malate; malonate; mevalonate	Malate is an intermediate in the citric acid cycle; malonate is a competitive inhibitor of the enzyme succinate dehydrogenase; mevalonate is an intermediate in cholesterol biosynthesis.
Melanin; melatonin	Melanin is the pigment of skin and hair; melatonin is a hormone synthesized by pineal gland.
Maltose; maltase	Maltose is a disaccharide; maltase is an enzyme that cleaves maltose to two molecules of glucose.
Methyl, methenyl; methylene	All the three are one-carbon fragments as shown in brackets, methyl ($-CH_3$); methenyl ($-CH=$); methylene ($-CH_2-$).
Molarity; molality	Molarity is defined as the number of moles of a solute per liter solution; molality represents the number of moles of a solute per 1,000 g of solvent.
Nicotinic acid; nicotine	Nicotinic acid is a β–complex vitamin; nicotine is an alkaloid present in tobacco leaves.
Nucleoside; nucleotide	A nucleoside is composed of a nitrogen base and a sugar; nucleotide contains one or more phosphate groups bound to nucleoside.

Term	Definition
Osmolarity; osmolality	Osmolarity represents osmotic pressure exerted by the number of moles (milli moles) per liter solution; osmolality refers to the osmotic pressure exterted by the number of moles (milli moles) per kg solvent.
Palmitate; palmitoleate	Both are even chain (16-carbon) fatty acids. Palmitate is a saturated fatty acid; palmitoleate is a monounsaturated fatty acid.
Phosphatidyl ethanolamine; phosphatidal ethanolamine	Both are phospholipids. In phosphatidyl ethanolamine, the fatty acid is bound by an ester linkage. The fatty acid is held by an ether linkage in phosphatidal ethanolamine.
Phytic acid; phytanic acid	Phytic acid is formed by the addition of six phosphate molecules to inositol, it is an inhibitor of the intestinal absorption of calcium and iron; phytanic acid is an unusal fatty acid derived from phytol, a constituent of chlorophyll.
Prokaryotes; eukaryotes	Prokaryotes are the cells that lack a well-defined nucleus; eukaryotes posses a well defined nucleus.
Prolamines; protamines	Both are simple proteins. Prolamines are soluble in alcohol; protamines are basic protein soluble in NH_4OH.
Pyridine; pyrimidine; pteridine	All the three are heterocyclic rings containing nitrogen, Pyridine ring is found in niacin and pyridoxine; pyrimidine is present in thiamine (vitamin B_1), thymine, cytosine and uracil; folic acid contains pteridine ring.
Pyridoxine; pyridoxal	Pyridine is the primary alcohol form of vitamin B_6; pyridoxal is the aldehyde form of B_6.
RDA; SDA	RDA (recommended dietary allowance) represents the quantities of nutrients to be provided in the diet daily for maintenance of good health and physical efficiency; specific dynamic action (SDA) is the extra heat produced by the body over and above the caloric value of foodstuffs.
Renin; Rennin	Renin is synthesized by the kidneys and is involved in vasoconstriction causing hypertension; rennin is an enzyme found in gastric juice responsible for coagulation of milk.

Term	Definition
Ribosomes; ribozymes	Ribosomes are the sites of protein biosynthesis; ribozymes refers to the RNA molecules which function as enzymes.
Retinol; retinal	Retinol is the alcohol form of vitamin A; retinal is the aldehyde form obtained by the oxidation of retinal.
Serotonin; melatonin	Serotonin is a neurotransmitter synthesized from tryptophan; melatonin is a hormone derived from serotonin in the pineal gland.
Somatotropin; somatostatin; somatomedin	Somatotropin is the other name for growth hormone (GH); growth release inhibiting hormone (GRIH) is also called somatostatin; somatomedin refers to the insulin-like growth factor-I (IGF-I), produced by liver in response to GH action.
Sucrose; sucrase	Sucrose is a disaccharide; sucrase is an enzyme that cleaves sucrose to glucose and fructose.
Synthase; synthetase	Both the enzymes are concerned with biosynthetic reactions. Synthase does not require ATP; synthetase is dependent on ATP for energy supply. (Note: most authors however, do not maintain this distinction between synthase and synthetase strictly).
Thiamine; thymine	Thiamine is a vitamin (B_1); thymine is a pyrimidine base found in DNA structure.
Thiokinase; thiolase	Thiokinase activates fatty acids to acyl CoA; Thiolase catalyses the final reaction in β–oxidation to liberate acetyl CoA from acyl CoA.
Transcription; translation	Transcription refers to the synthesis of RNA from DNA; translation involves the protein synthesis from the RNA.
Uric acid; uronic acid	Uric acid is the end product of purine metabolism; uronic acids are formed by the oxidation of aldehyde group of monsaccharides (e.g., glucuronic acid).
Ureotelic; uricotelic	Ureotelic organisms (e.g., mammals) convert NH_3 to urea; uricotelic organisms (e.g., reptiles) convert NH_3 to uric acid.
Vitamin A; coenzyme A	Vitamin A is fat-soluble vitamin; coenzyme A is derived from water-soluble vitamin, pantothenic acid.

9

NUTRITIONAL BIOCHEMICAL SHORT EXPLANATIONS

- Life is composed of lifeless chemical molecules. The complex biomolcules, proteins, nucleic acids (DNA and RNA), Polysaccharides and lipids are formed by the monomeric units amino acids, nucleotides, monosaccharides and fatty acids, respectively.

- The cell is the structural and functional unit of life. The eukaryotic cell consists of well-defined subcellular organelles, enveloped in a plasma membrane.

- The nucleus contains DNA, the repository of genetic information. DNA in association with proteins (histones) forms nucleosomes, which, in turn, make up the chromosomes.

- The mitochondria are the centers for energy metabolism. They are the principle producer of ATP, which is exported to all parts of the cell to provide energy for cellular work.

- Endoplasmic reticulum (ER) is the network of membrane-enclosed spaces that extends through the cytoplasm ER studded with ribosomes, the factories of protein biosynthesis is referred to as rough ER. Golgi apparatus is a cluster of membrane vesicles to which the newly synthesized proteins are handed over for future processing and export.

- Lysosomes are the digestive bodies of the cell, actively involved in the degradation of cellular compounds. Peroxisomes contain the enzyme catalase that protects the cell from the toxic effects of H_2O_2. The cellular ground matrix is referred to as filaments, the cytoskeleton.

- A living cell is a true representative of life with its own organization and specialized functions.

- Accumulation of lipofuscin, a pigment rich in lipids and proteins, in the cell has been implicated in ageing process.

- Leakage of lysosomal enzymes into the cell degrades several functional macromolecules and this may lead to certain disorders (e.g., arthritis).

- Carbohydrates are the polyhydroxyaldehydes or ketones or compounds, which produce them on hydrolysis. The term sugar is applied to carbohydrates soluble in water and sweet to taste.

- Carbohydrates are the major dietary energy sources, besides their involvement in cell structure and various other functions.

- Carbohydrates are broadly classified into 3 gropus-mono-saccharides, oligosaccharides and polysaccharides. The monosaccharides are further divided into different categories based on the presence of functional groups (aldoses or ketoses) and the number of carbon atoms (trioses, tetroses, pentoses, hexoses and heptoses).

- Glyceraldehyde (triose) is the simplest carbohydrate and is chosen as a reference to write the configuration of all other monosacchardies (D and L forms). If two monosaccharides differ in their structure around a single carbon atom, they are known as epimers, glucose and galactose are C_4 – epimers.

- D-Glucose is the most predominant naturally occurring aldose/ monosaccharide. Glucose exists as a and b anomers with different optical rotations. The inter conversion of a and b anomeric forms with change in the optical rotation is known as mutarotaion.

- Monosaccharides participate in several reactions. These include oxidation, reduction, dehydration, osazone formation etc. Formation of esters and glycosides by monosaccharides is of special significance in biochemical reactions.

- Among the oligosaccharides, disaccharides are the most common. These include the reducing disaccharides namely lactose (milk sugars) and maltose (malt sugar) and the non-reducing sucrose (cane sugar). Sucrose is dextrorotatory, but on hydrolysis it becomes levorotatory; this phenomenon is known as inversion.

- Polysaccharides are the polymer of monosaccharides or their derivatives, held together by glycosidic bonds. Homopolysaccharides are composed of a single monosaccharide (e.g., starch, glycogen, cellulose, insulin). Hetropolysaccharides contain a mixture of few monosaccharides or their derivatives (e.g., mucopolysaccharides).

- Starch and glycogen are the carbohydrate reserves of plants and animals respectively. Cellulose, exclusively found in plants, is the structural constituent. Insulin is utilized to assess kidney function by measuring glomerular filtration rate (GFR).

- Mucopolysaccharides (glycosaminoglycans) are the essential components of tissue structure. They provide the matrix or ground substance of extracellular tissue spaces in which collagen and elastin fibers are embedded. Hyaluronic acid, chondroitin 4-sulphate, heparin, are among the important glycosaminoglycans.

- Glycoproteins are a group of biochemically important compounds with a variable composition of carbohydrate (1-90%), covalently bound to proteins and cellular receptors are in fact glycoproteins. Anti freeze glycoproteins found in the Antarctic fish prevent the fish from being frozen.

- Glucose is the most important energy source of carbohydrates to the mammals (except ruminants). The bulk of dietary carbohydrate (starch) is digested and finally absorbed as glucose into the body.

- Lipids are the organic substances relatively insoluble in water, soluble in organic solvents (alcohol, ether, benzene, hexane) actually or potentially related to fatty acids and are utilized by the body.

- Lipids are classified into simple (fats and oils) complex (phospholipids) glycolipids, derived (fatty acids, steroid hormones) and miscellaneous (carotenoids).

- Fatty acids are the major constituents of various lipids. Saturated and unsaturated fatty acids almost equally occur in natural lipids. The polyunsaturated fatty acids (PUFA) namely linoleic acid and linolenic acid are the essential fatty acids that need to be supplied in the diet.

- Triacylglycerols (simply fats) are the esters of glycerol with fatty acids. They are found in adipose tissue and primarily function as fuel reserve of animals. Several tests (iodine number, RM number) are employed in the laboratory to test the purity of fats and oils.

- Phospholipids are complex lipids containing phosphoric acid. Glycerophospholipids contain glycerol as the alcohol and these include lecithin, cephalin, phosphatidylinositol, plasmalogen and cardiolipin.

- Sphingophospholipids (sphingo mycelins) contain sphingosine as the alcohol in place of glycerol (in glycerophospholipids). Phospholipids are the major constituents of plasma membranes.

- Cerebrosides are the simplest form of glycolipids, which occur in the membranes of nervous tissue. Gangliosides are predominantly found in the ganglions. They contain one or more molecules of N-acetylneuraminic acid (NANA).

- Steroids contain the ring cyclopentanoperhydrophenanthrene. The Steroids of biological importance include cholesterol, bile acids, vitamin D, sex hormones and cortical hormones. A steroid containing one or more hydroxyl groups is known as sterol.

- Cholesterol is the most abundant animal sterol. It contains one hydroxyl group (at C_3), a double bond ($C_5 - C_6$) and an eight-carbon side chain attached to C_{17}. Cholesterol is a constituent of membrane structure and is involved in the synthesis of bile acids, hormones (sex and cortical) and vitamin D.

- The lipids that possess both hydrophobic (non-polar) and hydrophilic (polar) groups are known as amphipathic. These include fatty acids, phospholipids, sphingolipids and bile salts. Amphipathic lipids are important constituents in the bilayers of the biological membranes.

- Proteins are nitrogen containing, most abundant organic macromolecules widely distributed in animals and plants. They perform structural and dynamic functions in the organisms.

- Proteins are polymers composed of L-α-amino acids. They are 20 in number and classified into different groups based on their structure, chemical nature, nutritional requirement and metabolic fate.

- Amino acids posses two functional groups namely carboxyl (-COOH) and ($-NH_2$). In the physiological system, they exist as dipolar ions commonly referred to as Zwitterions.

- Besides the 20 standard amino acids present in proteins, there are several non-standard amino acids. These include the amino acid derivatives found in proteins (e.g., hydoxy proline, hydroxylysine), non-protein amino acids (e.g., ornithine, citrulline) and D-amino acids.

- The structure of protein is divided into four levels of organization. The primary structure represents the linear sequence of amino acids. The twisting and special arrangement of polypeptide chain is the secondary structure. Tertiary structure constitutes the three-dimentional structure of a functional protein. The assembly of similar or dissimilar polypeptide subunits comprises quaternary structure.

- The determination of primary structure of a protein involves the knowledge of quality, quantity and the sequence of amino acids in the polypeptide. Chemical and enzymatic methods are employed for the determination of primary structure.

- The secondary structure of protein mainly consists of α–helix and/or β–Sheet. α–Helix is stabilized by extensive hydrogen bonding. β–Plated sheet is composed of two or more segments of fully extended polypeptide chains.

- Non-covalent bonds such as hydrogen bonds, hydrophobic interactions, ionic bonds etc. stabilize the tertiary and quaternary structures of proteins.

- Proteins are classified into three major groups. Simple proteins contain only amino acid residues (e.g., albumin). Conjugated proteins contain a non-protein moiety known as prosthetic group, besides the amino acids (e.g., glycoproteins). Derived proteins are obtained by degradation of simple or conjugated proteins.

- In addition to proteins, several peptides perform biologically important functions. These include glutathione, oxytocin and vasopressin.

- Vitamins are accessory food factors required in the diet. They are classified as fat-soluble (A, D, E and K) and water-soluble (B-complex and C).

- Vitamin A is involved in vision, proper growth, differentiation and maintenance of epithelial cells. Its deficiency results in night blindness.

- The active form of vitamin D is calcitriol which functions like a steroid hormone and regulates plasma levels of calcium and phosphate. Vitamin D deficiency leads to rickets in children and osteomalacia in adults.

- Vitamin E is a natural antioxidant necessary for normal reproduction in many animals.

- Vitamin K has a specific coenzyme function. It catalyses the carboxylation of glutamic acid residues in blood clotting factors (II, VIII, IX and X) and converts them to active form.

- Thiamine (B_1) as a coarboxylase (TPP) is involved in energy releasing reactions. Its deficiency leads to beriberi.

- The coenzymes of riboflavin (FAD and FMN) and niacin (NAD and NADP) take part in a variety of oxidation-reduction reactions connected with energy generation.

- Riboflavin deficiency results in cheilosis and glossitis whereas niacin deficiency leads to pellagra.

- Pyridoxal phosphate (PLP), the coenzyme of vitamin B_6, is mostly associated with amino acid metabolism. PLP participates in tansamination, decarboxylation, deamination and condensation reactions.

- Biotin (anti-egg white injury factor) participates as a coenzyme in carboxylation reactions of gluconeogenesis, fatty acid synthesis etc.

- Coenzyme A (of pantothenic acid) is involved in the metabolism of carbohydrates, lipids and amino acids and their integration.

- Tetrahydrofolate (THF), the coenzyme of folic acid participates in the transfer of one-carbon units (formyl, methyl etc.), in amino acid and nucleotide metabolism. Megaloblastic anemia is caused by folic acid deficiency.

- Vitamin B_{12} has two coenzymes, deoxyadenosylcobalamin and methylcobalamin. B_{12} deficiency results in pernicious anemia.

- Vitamin C (ascorbic acid) is involved in the hydroxylation of proline and lysine in the formation of collagen. Survey is caused by ascorbic acid deficiency.

- Therapeutic use of megadoses of vitamin C, to cure everything from use of cold to cancer, has become controversial.

- Certain vitamin like compounds (choline, inositol, PABA, lipoic acid) are also involved in many biochemical reactions.

- DNA is the chemical basis of heredity organized into genes, the basic units of genetic information.

- RNAs (mRNA, tRNA, and rRNA) are produced by DNA, which in turn carry out protein synthesis.

- Nucleic acids are the polymers of nucleotides (polynucleotides) held by 3' and 5' phosphodiester bridges. A nucleotide essentially consists of base + sugar (nucleoside) and phosphate.

- Besides being the constituents of nucleic acid structure, nucleotides perform a wide variety of cellular functions (e.g., energy carriers, metabolic regulators, second messengers).

- Both DNA and RNA contain the purines-adenine (A) and guanine (G) and the pyrimidine-Cytosine (C). The second pyrimidine is thymine (T) in DNA while it is uracil (U) in RNA.

- The pentose sugar, D-deoxyribose is found in DNA while it is D-ribose in RNA.

- The structure of DNA is a double helix (Watson-Crick model) composed of two antiparallel strands of polydeoxynucleotides twisted around each other. The strands are held together by 2 or 3 hydrogen bonds formed between the base i.e., A = T; G°C. DNA structure satisfies Chargaff's rule that the content of A is equal to T and that of G equal to C.

- RNA is usually a single strands polyribonucleotide. 7-methyl GTP while at the 3' -terminal end caps the mRNA at 5' terminal end; it contains a poly a tail. The mRNA specifies the sequence of amino acids in protein synthesis.

- The structure of tRNA resembles that of a colour leaf with four arms (acceptor, anticodon, D- and TYC) held by complementary base pairs, tRNA delivers amino acids for protein synthesis.

- RNAs (28s, 5s, 18s) are found in combination with proteins and are involved in the binding of mRNA to ribosomes and protein synthesis.

- Enzymes are the protein biocatalysts synthesized by the living cells. They are classified into six major classes-oxidoreductases, trnasferases, hydrolases, lyases, isomerases and ligases.

- An enzyme is specific in its action, possessing active site, where the substrate binds to form enzyme-substrate complex, before the product is formed.

- Factors like concentration of enzyme, substrate, temperature, and pH etc. influence enzyme activity. The substrate concentration to produce half-maximal velocity is known as Michaelis constant (Km value).

- Enzyme activities are inhibited by reversible (competitive, non-competitive and uncompetitive), irreversible and allosteric manner.

- Many enzymes require the presence of non-protein substances called cofactors (coenzymes) for their action. Most of the coenzymes are derivatives of B-complex vitamins (e.g., NAD^+, FAD, TPP etc.).

- The mechanism of enzyme action is explained by lock and key model (of Fisher), more recently induced fit model (of Koshland) and substrate strain theory.

  The enzymes enhance the rate of reaction through acid-base catalysis, covalent catalysis and or entropy effects.

- In the living system, there is a constant regulation of enzyme levels brought about by allosteric mechanism, activation of proenzymes, synthesis and degradation of enzymes etc.

- Estimation of serum enzymes is of great help in the diagnosis of several diseases. Serum amylase and lipase are increased in acute pancreatitis; alanine transaminase in hepatitis; aspartate transaminase; lactate dehydrogenase (LDH) and creative phosphotase in rickets and hyperparthyroidism; acid phosphatase in prostatic carcinoma; glutamyl transpeptidase in alcoholism.

- Isoenzymes are the multiple forms of an enzyme catalyzing the same reaction, which however, differ, in their physical and chemical properties. LDH has five isoenzymes while CPK has three. LDH and CPK are very important in the diagnosis of myocardial infarction.

- Digestion is a process that converts complex foodstuff into simpler ones, which can be readily absorbed by the gastro intestine tract.

- Stomach, duodenum and upper part of small intestine are the major sites of digestion. The small intestine is the prime site for the absorption of digested foods.

- The digestion of carbohydrates is initiated in the mouth by salivary α–amylase and is completed in the small intestine by pancreatic α–amylase, oligosaccharides and disaccharides.

- Monosaccharides are the final absorbable products of carbohydrate digestion. A carrier mediated transports glucose into the intestinal mucosal cells. Na^+ dependent energy requiring process.

- Lactose intolerance due to a defect in the enzyme lactase (β-galactosidase) resulting in the inability to hydrolyse lactose (milk sugar) is the common abnormality of carbohydrate digestion.

- Protein digestion beings in the stomach by pepsin, which is aided by gastric HCl. Pancreatic proteases (trypsin, chymotrypsin and elastase) and intestinal amino peptidases and dipeptidases compete the degradation of proteins to amino acids and some dipeptides.

- The intestinal absorption of amino acids occurs by different transport systems (at least six known). The uptake of amino acids is primarily a Na^+-dependent energy requiring process.

- Digestion of lipids occurs in the small intestines. Emulsification of lipids, brought about by bile salts, is a prerequisite for their digestion. Pancreatic lipase aided by a colipase degrades triacylglycerol to 2-monoacylglycerol and free fatty acids.

- Cholesterol esterase and phospholipases, respectively, hydrolyse cholesteryl esters and phospholipids.

- Lipid absorption occurs through mixed micelles, formed by bile salts in association with products of lipid digestion (primarily 2-monoacylglycerol, cholesterol and free fatty acids). In the intestinal mucosal cells, lipids are resynthesized from the absorbed components and packed as chylomicrons, which enter the lymphatic vessels and then the blood.

- Dietary nucleic acids (DNA and RNA) are digested in the small intestine to nucleosides and/or bases (purines and pyrimidines), which are absorbed.

- The total concentration of plasma proteins is about 6-8 g/dl. Electrophoresis separates plasma proteins into 5 distinct bonds, namely albumin α_1, α_2, β and globulins.

- Albumin is the major constituent (60%) of plasma proteins with a concentration 3.5 to 5.0 g/dl. It is exclusively synthesized in the liver. Albumin performs osmotic, transport and nutritive functions.

- α_1 -Antitrypsin is a major constituent of α_1–globulin fraction. α_1–Antitrypsin deficiency has been implicated in emphysema and a specific liver disease.

- Haptoglobulin (HP) binds with free hemoglobin (Hb) that spills into the plasma due to hemolysis. The Hp-Hb complex cannot pass through the glomeruli; hence haptoglobin prevents the loss of free hemoglobin into urine.

- Immunoglobulins are specialized proteins to defend the body against the foreign substances. They are mostly associated with r-globulin fraction of plasma proteins. The immunoglobulin essentially consists of two identical heavy chains and two identical light chains, held together by disulfide linkages.

- Five classes of immunoglobulins namely IgG, IgA, IgM, IgD and IgE are found in humans. IgG is most abundant and is mainly responsible for humoral immunity. IgA protects body surfaces. IgM serves as a first line of defense for humoral immunity while IgE is associated with allergic reactions.

- Multiple myeloma is due to the malignancy of a single clone of plasma cells in the bone marrow. This causes the overproduction of abnormal IgG. The plasma of multiple myeloma patients on electrophoresis shows a distinct M-band.

- The complement system is composed of about 20 plasma proteins that complement the functions of antibodies in defending the body from invading antigens. The complement system helps the body immunity in several ways-promoting phagocytosis, clearance of antigen-antibody complexes etc.

- Blood clotting is the body's major defense mechanism against blood loss. The extrinsic and intrinsic pathways lead to the formation of factor Xa, which then participates in the final common pathway to active prothrombin to thrombin. Fibrinogen is then converted to fibrin clot.

- Plasmin is mostly responsible for the dissolution of fibrin clots. Plasminogen, synthesized by the kidney, is the inactive precursor of plasmin. Tissue plasminogen activator (TPA) and urokinase convert plasminogen to plasmin.

- Hemoglobin (HbA_1, mol. Wt. 64,450) is a conjugated protein containing globulin, the apoprotein and the heme, the non-protein moiety (prosthetic group). It is a tetrameric, allosteric protein with 2a and 2b polypeptide chains held by non-covalent interactions. Each subunit contains a heme with iron in the ferrous state.

- Hemoglobin is responsible for the transport of O_2 from lungs to the tissues. Each heme (of Hb) can bind with one molecule of O_2 and this is facilitated by cooperative heme-heme interaction.

- Hemoglobin activity participates in the transport of CO_2 from tissues to lungs. Increased partial pressure of CO_2 ($P\,CO_2$) accompanied by elevated H^+ decreases the binding of O_2 to Hb, a phenomenon known as Bohr effect.

- The four compounds namely 2,3-bisphosphoglycerate, CO_2, H^+ and Cl^- are collectively known as allosteric effectors. They interact with hemoglobin and facilitate the release of O_2 from oxyHb.

- Sickle-cell anemia (Hbs) is a classical example of abnormal hemoglobin's. It is caused when glutamate at 6th position of B-chain is replaced by valine. Hbs is characterized by hemolytic anemia, tissue damage, increased susceptibility to infection and premature death. Sickle cell anemia, however offers resistance to malaria.

- Thalassemias are a group of hereditary hemolytic disorders characterized by impairment/imbalance in the synthesis of globin (α or β) chain of Hb. Hydrops fetalis, the most severe form of α–thalassemia is characterized by the death of infant at birth. β–Thalassemia major is another serious disorder with severe anemia and death of child within 1–2 years.

- Heme is the most important porphyrin compound, primarily synthesized in the liver from the presusors-glycine and succinyl CoA. Heme production is regulated by δ–aminolevulinate synthase.

- Porphyrias are the metabolic disorders of heme synthesis, characterized by the increased excretion of porphyrins or their precursors. Acute intermittent porphyria occurs due to the deficiency of the enzyme uroporphyrinogen I synthase and is characterized by increased excretion of porphobilinogen and δ–aminolevulinate. The clinical symptoms include neuropsychiatric disturbances and cardiovascular abnormalities.

- Heme is degraded mainly to bilirubin, a yellow colour bile pigment. In the liver, it is conjugated to bilirubin diglucuronide, a more easily excreatable form into bile.

- Jaundice is a clinical condition caused by elevated serum bilirubin concentration (normal < 0.8 mg/dl). Jaundice is of three types-hemolytic (due to increased hemolysis), hepatic (due to impaired conjugation) and obstructive (due to obstruction in the bile duct).

- Bioenergetics deals with the study of energy changes in biochemical reactions. Changes in free energy (ΔG) are valuable in predicting the feasibility of a reaction. A negative and a positive ΔG, respectively, represent an exergonic (energy-releasing) and endergonic (energy-consuming) reaction.

- High energy compounds ($\Delta G > -7.0$ cal/mol) play a crucial role in the energy transfer of biochemical reactions (e.g., ATP, phosphocreatine, phosphoenol pyruvate).

- ATP is the energy currency of the cell. ATP-ADP cycle acts as a connecting energy link between catabolic and anabolic reactions.

- Respiratory chain or electron transport chain (ETC) located in the inner mitochondrial membrane represents the final stage of oxidizing the reducing equivalents (NADH and $FADH_2$) derived from the metabolic intermediates to water.

- ETC is organized into five distinct complexes. The complexes I to IV are electron carriers while complex V is responsible for ATP production. The components of ETC are arranged in the sequence.
  NAD^+ FMN $\longrightarrow$ CoQ $\longrightarrow$ Cytb $\longrightarrow$ Cytc$_1$ $\longrightarrow$ Cytc $\longrightarrow$ Cyta + a$_3$ $\longrightarrow$ O_2.

- The process of synthesizing ATP from ADP and Pi coupled with ETC is known as oxidative phosphorylation. NADH oxidation with P:O ratio 3 indicates that 3 ATP are synthesized while $FADH_2$ oxidation (P:O ratio 2) results in the production of 2 ATP.

- Among the hypothesis put forth to explain the mechanism of oxidative phosphorylation, the chemiosmotic hypothesis (of Mitchell) is widely accepted. The flow of electrons through the ETC causes proton (H^+) gradient across the inner mitochondrial, membrane, which leads to the synthesis of ATP from ADP and Pi, catalyzed by ATP synthetase.

- NADH produced in the cytosol cannot directly enter in to mitochondria. Glycerol-phosphate shuttle (generates 2 ATP) and malate-asparate shuttle (generate 3 AATP) operate to overcome the difficulty.

- There are many inhibitors of electron transport chain (rotenone, amytal, antimycin, CO-CN, H_2S etc) and oxidative phosphorylation (oligomycin, atractyloside). Uncouplers (e.g., dinitrophenol) are the substances the delink ETC from oxidative phosphorylation.

  Free radicals are chemicals species that posses one or more unpaired electrons (O_2^-, H_2O_2, OH^-) that have been implicated in the causation of several diseases (cancer, inflammatory diseases, cataract). The body, however, has a defense mechanism in the form of antioxidant system (superoxide dismutase, catalase) to scavenger free radicals.

- The wide range of chemical reactions occurring in the living system is collectively known as metabolism. Catabolism is concerned with the degradation of complex molecules to simpler ones coupled with the liberation of energy (ATP). On the other hand, anabolism deals with the synthetic reactions converting simple precursors to complex molecules, coupled with the consumption of energy (ATP). A metabolic pathway constitutes a series of enzymatic reactions to produce specific products.

- Several methods are employed to study metabolism. These include the use of the whole organism or its components (organ, tissue, cells, organelles etc.), utility of metabolic probes (inhibitors and mutations) and application of isotopes.

- Carbohydrates are the major sources of energy for the living cells. Glucose (normal fasting blood level 70–100 mg/dl) is the central molecule in carbohydrate metabolism, actively participating in a number of metabolic pathways glycolysis, gluconeogenesis, glycogenesis, glycogenolysis, hexose monophosphate shunt, uronic acid pathway etc.

- Glucose is oxidized in glycolysis, either in anaerobic (2ATP formed) or aerobic (8 ATP formed) conditions, resulting in the formation of 2 moles of lactate or pyruvate, respectively.

- Acetyl CoA is produced from pyruvate, which is completely oxidized in citric acid cycle, the final common oxidative pathway for all foodstuffs. The complete oxidation of one mole of glucose generates 38 ATP.

- Gluconeogenesis is the synthesis of glucose from noncarbohyrate precursors like amino acids (except leucine and lysine), lactate, glycerol, propionate etc. The reversal of glycolysis with alternate arrangements made at three irreversible reactions of glycolysis constitutes gluconeogenesis.

- Glycogen is the storage form of glucose. The degradation of glycogen (glycogenolysis) in muscles the immediate fuel requirements, whereas the liver glycogen maintains the blood glucose level. Enzyme defects in synthesis or degradation of glycogen lead to storage disorders. Von Gierke's disease (Type I) is due to the defect in the enzyme glucose 6-phosphatase.

- Hexose monophosphate shunt (HMP shunt) is the direct oxidative pathway of glucose. HMP shunt assumes significance since it generates NADPH and pentoses, respectively required for the synthesis of lipids and nucleic acids.

- Glucuronate involved in the conjugation of bilirubin, steroid hormones and detoxification of drugs is synthesized in uronic acid pathway. Due to a single enzyme defect (gulonolactone oxidase) in this pathway, man cannot synthesize ascorbic acid (Vitamin C) whereas some animals can.

- Galactosemia is mostly due to the defect in the enzyme galactose 1-phosphate uridyltransferase. This results in the diversion of galactose to produce galactitol, which has been implicated in the development of cataract.

- Glucose can be converted to fructose via sorbitol pathway. In prolonged hyperglycemia (uncontrolled diabetes), sorbitol accumulates in the tissues, resulting in cataract, nephropathy, peripheral neuropathy etc.

  Amino sugars (glucosamine, galactosamine, mannosamine etc.), synthesized from fructose 6-phosphate are essential components of glycosaminoglycans, glycolipids and glycoproteins.

- Triacylglycerols (TG) are the highly concentrated from of energy, stored in adipose tissue. Hormone-sensitive lipase hydrolysis TG to free fatty acids, which are transported as albumin-FFA complexes.

- Fatty acids are activates (acyl CoA) and transported by carnitine to mitochondria where they get oxidized (mostly β type) to liberate energy. Complete oxidation of one mole palmitate liberates 129 ATP.

- Excessive utilization of fatty acids occurs in uncontrolled diabetes mellitus and starvation. This results in the overproduction of ketone bodies (in liver), namely acetone, acetoacetic acid and β–hydroxy butyric acid. The last two ketone bodies serve as energy source for peripheral tissues.

- Fatty acid biosynthesis occurs from acetyl CoA in the cytosol through the involvement of a multienzyme complex associated with acyl carrier protein (ACP). The reducing equivalents (NADPH + H$^+$) are supplied mostly by HMP shunt.

- Synthesis of triacylglycerols and phospholipids (PL) occurs from glycerol 3-phosphoate and dihydroxyacetate phosphate with the addition of acyl CoA, and activated nitrogenous bases (for PL).

- Cholesterol is synthesized from acetyl CoA in a series of reactions involving HMG CoA, mevalonate, isopernoid units and squalene as the intermediates. Cholesterol serves as a precursor for bile acids, steroid hormones and vitamin D.

- Lipoproteins are the transport vehicles for lipids in the plasma. Lipoprotein disorders are associated with abnormalities in their plasma levels. Elevation in LDL and VLDL in association with cholesterol and TG-poses a serious health problem with increased risk of atherosclerosis and CHD (coronary heart disease).

- Excessive accumulation of triacylglycerols in liver causes fatty liver, which may be due to increased production of TG or impairment in lipoprotein (VLDL) synthesis. The latter is mostly associated with the deficiency of certain substances called lipotropic factors (e.g., choline, betaine, methionine etc.).

- Obesity is an abnormal increase in body weight (with more than 25% due to fat). Among the many causative factors of obesity, lack of active brown adipose tissues (which burn fat and liberate heat) in these individuals is gaining importance.

- Atherosclerosis is a complex disease characterized by thickening of arteries due to the accumulation of lipids. Atherosclerosis and coronary heart disease (CHD) are directly correlated with LDL and inversely with HDL of plasma.

- The body proteins are in a dynamic state (degradation and synthesis) and there is an active amino acid pool (100 g) maintained for this purpose.

- The amino acids undergo transamination and deamination to liberate ammonia for the synthesis of urea the end product of protein metabolism.

- Besides being present as structural components of proteins, amino acids participate in the formation of several biologically important compounds.

- Glycine is involved in the synthesis of creatine, heme purines, glutathione etc.

- Phenylalanine is hydroxylated to tyrosine, which is a precursor for the production of skin pigment (melanin), catecholamines (dopamine, epinephrine and norepinephrine) and thyroid hormones (T$_3$ and T$_4$).

- Trptophan is converted to NAD^+ and $NADP^+$ the coenzyme of niacin, serotonin (a neurotransmitter) and melatonin.

- The active methionine (SAM) is a donor of methyl group (transmethylation) for the synthesis of many biological compounds (epinephrine, choline, methyl cytosine etc.).

- Many amino acids contribute to one carbon fragments (formyl, formimino, methylene etc.) for participation in one carbon metabolism, which is mostly under the control of tetrhydrofolate.

- The carbon skeleton of amino acids is involved either in the synthesis of glucose (glycogenic) or fat (ketogenic) or both glucose and fat.

- Many inborn errors (mostly due to enzyme defects) in amino acid metabolism have been identified. These include phenylketonuria (defect-phenylalanine hydroxylase), albinism (defect-tyrosine), maple syrup urine disease (defect-α-keto acid dehydrogenase) etc.

- The metabolism of carbohydrates, lipids and proteins is integrated to meet the energy and metabolic demands of the organism. The metabolic pathways-glycolysis, fatty acid oxidation, citric acid cycle and oxidative phosphorylation are directly concerned with the generation of ATP, Gluconeogesis, glycogen metabolism, hexose monophosphate shunt and amino acid degradation are also associated with energy metabolism.

- The organs/tissues, with their respective specializations, coordinate with each other to meet the metabolic demands of the organism as a whole. Liver is specialized to serve as the body's central metabolic clearinghouse. It processes and distributes the nutrients to different tissues for their utilization. Adipose tissue is primarily a storage organ of fat. The major bulk of the body protein is located in the muscle tissue.

- Brain is a specialized organ, which, in the normal situation, is exclusively dependent on the supply of glucose (120 g/day) for its fuel needs.

- Starvation is a metabolic stress, as it imposes certain metabolic compulsions on the organism. The stored fat of adipose tissue and the muscle protein are degraded and utilized to meet the body's fuel demands. Brain gradually adopts itself to use ketone bodies (instead of glucose) for its energy requirements. Starvation is thus associated with metabolic reorganization for the survival of the organism.

- Nucleotides participate in a wide variety of reactions in the living cells-synthesis of DNA and RNA; as constituents of many coenzymes; in the regulation of metabolic reactions etc.

- Purine nucleotides are synthesized in a series of reactions starting from ribose 5-phosphate. Glucose, gluctamine, aspartate, formate and CO_2 contribute to the synthesis of purine ring.

- Purine nucleotides can also be synthesized from free purines by a salvage pathway. The defect in the enzyme HGPRT causes Lesch-Nyham syndrome.

- Deoxyribonucleotides are formed from ribonucleotides by a reduction process catalyzed by ribonucleotide reductase. Thioredoxin is the protein cofactor required for this reaction.

- Purine nucleotides are degraded to uric acid, the excretory product in humans. Uric acid serves as a natural antioxidant in the living system.

- Uric acid in many animal species (other than primates) is converted to more soluble forms such as allantoin, allantoic acid etc. and excreted.

- Gout is a metabolic disease associated with overproduction of uric acid. This often leads to the accumulation of sodium urate crystals in the joints, causing painful gouty arthritis. Allopurinol, an inhibitor of xanthine oxidase is the drug used for the treatment of gout.

- Pyrimidine nucleotides are synthesized from the precursors aspartate, glutamine and CO besides ribose 5-phosphate.

- Orotic aciduria is a defect in pyrimidine synthesis caused by the deficiency of orotate phosphoribosyltranferase and OMP decarboxylase. Diet rich in uridine and/or cytidine is an effective treatment for orotic aciduria.

- Pyrimidines are degraded to amino acids, namely β–alanie and β–aminoisobutyrate, which are then metabolized.

- The central dogma of life revolves around the flow of information from DNA to RNA and from there to protein. It is ultimately DNA that controls energy cellular function.

- Replication is a process in which DNA copies itself to produce identical daughter molecules of DNA. DNA synthesis is semi conservative, bi-directional and occurs by the formation of bubbles and forks. Replication requires RNA primer and DNA polymerase III. The new DNA is produced as small fragments (okazaki pieces) are joined together by DNA ligases.

- Transcription is a process in which RNA is synthesized from DNA, which is carried out in 3 stages initiation, elongation and termination. The enzyme RNA polymerase binds to the promoter region of DNA and the transcription proceeds in 5′ $\longrightarrow$ 3′ direction (antiparallel to DNA template) till it is stopped by the termination signals.

- In case of eukaryotes, RNA polymerases I, II and III respectively catalyze the formation of rRNAs, mRNAs and tRNAs.

- Biosynthesis of a protein or a polypeptide is known as translation. The amino acid sequence of a protein is determined by the triplet nucleoside base sequence of mRNA, arranged as codons or genetic code.

- The genetic code-composed of A, G, C and U is universal, unambiguous, nonoverlapping and degenerate of the 64 codons, three (UAA, UAG, and UGA) are termination codons, while the rest 61 code for amino acids.

- The process of translation involves activation of amino acids followed by initiation, elongation and termination of protein synthesis.

- Ribosomes are the factories of protein biosynthesis. The inhibition factors (IF_1, IF_2 and IF_3), mRNA and tRNA (with amino acid) bind to 30s ribosome which then form 70s complex by a sequential addition of amino acids (supplied by tRNAs) as determined by codons of mRNA. The peptide bonds hold the amino acids together and the growing polypeptide chain is terminated by stop signals (terminating codons) guided by release factor (RF-1, RF-2 and RF-3).

- Several antibiotics such as streptomycin, tetracyclines, puromycin and chloramphenicol inhibit translation.

- The modifications that occur in the protein after it is synthesized are collectively known as post-translational modifications. These include the proteolytic degradation and covalent modifications (phosphorylation, hydroxylation, glycosylation etc.).

- Mutation refers to a change in the DNA structure of gene. The alterations that occur in the DNA are reflected in replication, transcription and translation.

- The minerals or inorganic elements are required for normal growth and maintenance of the body. They are classified as principal elements and trace elements. These are seven principal elements Ca, P, Mg, Na, K, Cl, F, Se and Cr.

- Calcium is required for the development of bones and teeth, muscle contraction, blood coagulation, nerve transmission etc. Vitamin D, PTH and acidity promote absorption of Ca from the duodenum while it is inhibited by phytate, oxalate, free fatty acids and fiber. The normal level of serum Ca (9 – 11 mg/dl) is controlled by interplay of PTH, calcitriol and calcitonin.

- Serum Ca levels elevated in hyperparathyroidism and diminished in hypoparathyroidism. Hypocalcemia causes tetany, the symptoms of which include neuromuscular irritability, spasm and convulsions.

- Phosphorus, besides being essential for the development of bones and teeth, is a constituent of high-energy phosphate compounds (ATP, GTP) and nucleotide coenzymes (NAD^+, $NADP^+$).

- Sodium, potassium and chlorine are involved in the regulation of acid-base equilibrium, fluid balance and osmotic pressure in the body. Sodium is the principal extracellular cation (serum level 135 – 145 mEq/L), while potassium is the chief intracellular cation (serum level 3.5 - 5.0 mEq/L).

- Iron is mainly required for O_2 transport and cellular respiration. Absorption of iron is promoted by ascorbic acid, cysteine, acidity and small peptides while it is inhibited by phytate, oxalate and high phosphate.

- Iron (Fe^{+++}) is transported in the plasma in a bound form to transferring. It is stored as ferritin in liver, spleen and bone marrow. Iron deficiency anemia causes microcytic hypochromic anemia. Excessive consumption of iron results in hemosiderosis, which is due to the tissue deposition of hemosiderin.

- Copper is an essential constituent of several enzymes (e.g., Catalase, cytochrome oxidase, tyrosinase). Ceruloplasmin is a copper containing protein required for the transport of iron (Fe^{+++}) in the plasma. Wilson's disease is an abnormality in copper metabolism, characterized by the deposition of copper in liver, brain and kidney.

- Iodine is important as a component of thyroid hormones (T_4 and T_3) while cobalt is a constituent of Vitamin B_{12}. Zinc is necessary for the storage and secretion of insulin and maintenance of normal vitamin A levels in serum, besides being a component of several enzymes (e.g., carbonic anhydrase, alcohol dehydrogenase).

- Fluorine in trace amounts (2 ppm) prevents dental caries while its higher intake leads to fluorosis. Selenium is assigned an antioxidant role as it protects the cells from free radicals. Chromium promotes the utilization of glucose and reduces serum cholesterol.

- Hormones are the organic substances, produced in minute quantities by specific tissues (endocrine glands) and secreted into the blood stream to control the biological activities in the target cells. They may be regulated as the chemical messengers involved in the regulation and coordination of body functions.

- Hormones are classified based on their chemical nature or mechanism of action. Chemically, they may be proteins or peptides (insulin, oxytocin), steroids (glucocorticoids, sex hormones) and amino acid derivatives (epinephrine, thyroxin). By virtue of the function, group I hormones bind to the intracellular receptors (estrogens, calcitriol), while group II hormones (ACTH, LH) bind to the cell surface receptors and act through the second messengers.

- Cyclic (cAMP) is an intracellular second messenger for a majority of polypeptide hormones. Membrane bound adenylate cyclase enzyme, through the mediation of G proteins is responsible for the synthesis of cAMP. CAMP acts through protein kinases that phosphorylate specific proteins, which, in turn, causes the ultimate biochemical response. Phosphatidylinositol/calcium system also functions as a second messenger for certain hormones (TRH, gastrin).

- Hypothalamus is the master coordinator of hormonal action as it liberates certain releasing factors or hormones (TRH, CRH, GRH, GRIH) that stimulate or inhibit the corresponding trophic hormones from the anterior pituitary.

- Anterior pituitary gland is the master endocrine organ that produces several hormones which influences either directly or indirectly (through the mediation of other endocrine organs) a variety of biochemical processes in the body. For instance, growth hormone is directly involved in growth promoting process while TSH, FSH and ACTH, respectively influences thyroid gland, gonads and adrenal cortex to synthesize hormones.

- Thyroid gland produces two principal hormones-thyroxin (T4) and triodothyronine (T_3), which are primarily concerned with the regulation of the metabolic activity of the body. Goiter is a disorder caused by enlargement of thyroid gland and is mainly due to iodine deficiency in the diet.

- Adrenal cortex synthesizes glucocorticoids (e.g., cortisol) that influence glucose, amino acid and fat metabolism, and mineral corticoids (e.g., aldosterone) that regulate water and electrolyte balance. Androgens and estrogen (sex hormones) in small quantities are also synthesized by the adrenal cortex.

- Adrenal medulla produces two important hormones, epinephrine and nor epinephrine (catecholamines). They influence diversified biochemical functions with an ultimate goal to mobilize energy resources and prepare the individual to meet emergencies (shock, anger, fatigue etc.).

- The testes and ovaries respectively synthesize the steroid sex hormones, primarily androgens in males and estrogens in females. These hormones are responsible for growth, development, maintenance and regulation of reproductive system in either sex.

- Several gastrointestinal hormones (e.g., gastrin, secretin) have been identified that are closely involved in the regulation of digestion and absorption of foodstuffs.

- Specific laboratory biochemical investigations are employed to assess the functioning of the organs such as liver, kidney, stomach and pancreas.

- The liver functions can be elevated by the tests based on its excretory function (serum bilirubin), serum enzymes (transaminases), metabolic capacity (galactose tolerance test) and synthetic functions (prothrombin time).

- Water is the solvent of life and constituents about 60% of the total body weight, distributed in intracellular and extracellular fluids. The daily water intake (by drinking, from foodstuff and metabolic water) and out put (loss via urine, skin, lungs and feces) maintain the body balance of water.

- Electrolytes are distributed in the intracellular and extracellular fluids to maintain the osmotic equilibrium and water balance; Na^+ is the principal extracellular cation while K^+ is the intracellular cation. As regards anions, Cl^- and HCO_3^- predominantly occur in the extracellular fluids while HPO_4^-, proteins and organic acids are present in the intracellular fluids.

- The osmolality of plasma is about 285 milliosmoles/kg, which is predominantly contributed by Na^+ and its associated anions. Thus, for practical purposes, plasma osmolality can be calculated from Na^+ concentration ($2 \times Na^+$ in mmol/L).

- Water and electrolyte balance are usually regulated together and this is under the control of hormones aldosterone, antidiuretic hormone and rennin.

- Dehydration of the body may be due to insufficient water intake or its excessive loss or both. Depletion of water in the ICF causes disturbance in metabolism. The manifestations of severe dehydration include increased pulse rate, low blood pressure, sunken eyeballs, decreased skin turgor, lethargy and coma.

- The normal pH of blood is maintained in the narrow range of 7.35 – 7.45. The metabolism of the body is accompanied by an overall production of acids. The body has developed three lines of defense (blood buffers, respiratory and renal mechanisms) to regulate the acid-base balance and maintain the blood pH.

- Among the blood buffers, bicarbonate buffer (with a ratio of HCO_3^- to H_2CO_3 as 20:1) is the most important in regulating blood pH. Phosphate and protein buffer systems also contribute in this regard. The respiratory system regulates the concentration of carbonic acid by controlling the elimination of CO_2 via lungs.

- The renal (kidney) mechanism regulates blood pH by excreting H^+ and NH_4^+ ions besides the reabsorption of HCO_3^-. The pH of urine is normally acidic which indicates that the kidneys have contributed to the acidification of urine.

- The acid-base disorders are classified as acidosis (metabolic or respiratory) and alkalosis (metabolic or respiratory), respectively, due to a rise or fall in blood pH. The metabolic disturbances are associated with alternations in HCO_3^- concentration while the respiratory disorders are due to changes in H_2CO_3 (i.e., CO_2).

- The difference between the total concentrations of measured cations (Na^+ and K^+) and that of measured anions (Cl^- and HCO_3^-) is referred to anion gap (normal around 15 mEq/L). The anion gap is increased in metabolic acidosis as is observed in severe uncontrolled diabetes mellitus.

- Serum bilirubin (normal < 1 mg/dl) is derived from heme degradation. It is mostly (75 % found in the conjugated form Van den Bergh reaction is a specific test to identify the increased serum bilirubin. Conjugated bilirubin gives a direct positive test while the unconjaguated bilirubin gives an indirect positive test.

- The serum enzymes-namely alanine transaminase (ALT), asparate transaminase (AST), alkaline phosphatase (ALP) and γ–glutamyltranspeptidase (GGT) are frequently used for LFT. Increase in the activities of these enzymes indicates impairment in liver function.

- Jaundice is due to elevated serum bilirubin level (> 2 mg/dl). The three types of jaundice (hemolytic obstructive and hepatic) can be differentially diagnosed by biochemical tests. Thus unconjugated bilirubin (indirect positive) is increased in hemolytic jaundice, conjugated bilirubin (direct positive) in obstructive jaundice and both of them (biphasic) are increased in hepatic jaundice.

- Impaired galactose tolerance test, diminished serum albumin concentration and prolonged prothrombin time are also associated with liver malfunction.

- The renal (kidney) function is usually assessed by evaluation either the glomerular (clearance tests) or tubular function (urine concentration test). This is often guided by blood analysis (for urea, creatinine) and/or urine examination.

- The clearance is defined as the volume of the plasma that would be completely cleared of a substance per minute. Insulin clearance represents glomerular filtration rate (GFR). Creatinine clearance and urea clearance tests are often used to assess venal function. A decrease in their clearance is an indication of renal damage.

- Impairment in renal function is often associated with elevated concentration of blood urea, serum creatinine, decrease in osmolality and specific gravity of urine (by urine concentration test).

- The tests to evaluate gastric function include fractional test meal, pentagastrin stimulation test, augmented histamine test and tubeless gastric analysis. Gastric HCl secretion is elevated in chronic duodenal ulcer and gastric hyperplasma. Gastritis and pancrriicious anemia are associated with decreased gastric HCl. Pancreatic function is assessed by serum amylase and lipase. Both of them are elevated in acute pancreatitis.

- The calorific values of carbohydrates, fats and proteins respectively are 4, 9 and 4 Cal/g. These three nutrients (macronutrients) supply energy to the body to meet the requirements of basal metabolic rate, specific dynamic action and physical activity.

- Basal metabolic rate (BMR) represents the minimum amount of energy required by the body to maintain life at complete physical and mental rest, in the post-absorptive state. The normal BMR for an adult man is $35 - 38$ Cal/m^2 body surface/hr.

- Specific dynamic action (SDA) is the extra heat produced by the body over and above the calculated calorific value of foodstuff. It is, higher for proteins (30%), lower for carbohydrate (5%) and for a mixed diet, it is around 10%.

- Carbohydrates are the major source of body fuel supplying about $40 - 70\%$ of body calories. The non-digested carbohydrates (cellulose, pectin) are refereed to as fiber. Adequate intake of fiber prevents constipation, improves glucose tolerance and reduces plasma cholesterol.

- Lipids are the concentrated source of energy. They also provide essential fatty acids (linoleic and linolenic acids) and fat-soluble vitamins (A, D, E and K).

- Proteins are the body building foods that supply essential amino acids, besides meeting the body energy requirement partly (10- 15%).

- Several methods are employed to assess the nutritive value of proteins. These include protein efficiency ratio, biological value, net protein utilization and chemical score.

- The recommended dietary allowance (RDA) represents the quantities of nutrients to be provided daily in the diet for maintaining good health and physical efficiency. The RDA for protein is 1 g/kg body weight/day.

- A balanced diet is the diet, which contains different types of foods with the nutrients, namely carbohydrates, fats, proteins, vitamins, and minerals; in a proportion to meet the body requirements.

- Protein-energy malnutrition (PEM) is the most common nutritional disorder in the developing countries. Kwashiorkor is primarily due to the inadequate protein intake while marasmus is mainly caused by calorie deficiency.

- Detoxification deals with the series of biochemical reactions occurring in the body to convert the foreign (often toxic) compounds to non-toxic or less toxic and more easily excretable forms. Liver is the major site of detoxification. In recent years, the term detoxification is replaced by biotransformation or metabolism of xenobiotics.

- Detoxification may be divided into phase I (oxidation, reduction, hydrolysis) and phase II reactions (conjugation). Oxidation is major process of detoxification, involving the microsomal enzyme cytochrome $P_{450,}$ which is an inducible, NADPH dependent hemoprotein.

- Conjugation is a process in which a foreign compound combines with a substrate produced in the body. The process of conjugation may occur either directly or after phase I reactions. At least 8 different conjugating agents have been identified in the body-gluconic acid, glycine, cysteine, glutamne, methyl group, sulfate, acetic acid and thiosulfate.

- Prostaglandins (PGs) and related compounds prostacyclins (PGI), thromboxanes (TXA) and leukotrienes (LT) are collectively known as eicosanoids. They are the derivatives of a hypothetical 20-carbon fatty acid, namely prostanoic acid. Prostaglandins are synthesized from arachidonic acid, released from the membrane bound phospholipids. Corticosteroids and aspirin inhibit PG synthesis.

- Prostaglandins act as loca hormones and are involved in a wide range of biochemical functions. In general, PGs are involved in the lowering of blood pressure, induction of inflammation, medical termination of pregnancy, induction of labor, inhibition of gastric HCl secretion, decrease in immunological response and increase in glomerular filtration rate. Thromboxanes (TXA_2) and prostaglandin E_1 promote while prostacyclins (PGI_2) inhibit platelet aggregation.

- Due to their diversified functions, PGs have been exploited for therapeutic use. They are utilized for the treatment of gastric ulcers, hypertension, thrombosis, asthma, medical termination of pregnancy, induction of labor etc. Inhibitors of PG synthesis (aspirin, ibuprofen) are used in controlling fever, pain, migraine, inflammation etc.

- Certain fish foods contain an unsaturated fatty acid, namely eicosapentaenoic acid (EPA) that inhibits the synthesis of TXA_2. Low levels of TXA_2 reduce platelet aggregation and thrombosis and therefore, lower the incidence of heart attacks. Thus, consumption of EPA is related to reduce risk myocardial complications.

- The biological membranes are the barrier that protects the cell and the sub cellular organelles from the hostile environment. The membranes are primarily composed of a lipid bilayer onto which the globular proteins are irregularly embedded to form a fluid mosaic model.

- Transport of molecules through membranes occurs either by passive diffusion, facilitated diffusion or active transport. Active transport occurs against a concentration gradient, which is dependent on the supply of metabolic energy (ATP). $Na^+ - K^+$ pump is responsible for the maintenance of high K^+ and low Na^+ concentrations inside the cells, an essential requisite for the survival of cells.

- The transport of macromolecules takes place by endocytosis (ingestion by the cells) and exocytosis (release from the cells).

- DNA the chemical vehicle of heredity is composed of functional units-genes. The regulation of gene expression is absolutely essential for the growth, development and differentiation of an organism. A positive regulator increases the gene expression whereas a negative regulator decreases.

- The operon is the coordinated unit of genetic expression in bacteria. The lac operon of *E. coli* consists of regulatory genes and structural genes. The lac repressor binds to the DNA and halts the process of transcription of the structural genes. However, the pressure of lactose inactivates the repressor (depression) leading to the expression of structural genes. A catabolite gene activator protein (CAP) in association with cAMP is also involved in the transcription of lac operon.

- The expression of eukaryotic genes is very complex, involving several mechanisms. These include gene amplification, gene rearrangement and synthesis, transport, processing and stability of mRNA. The process of gene rearrangement is responsible for the generation of 10 billions (10^{10}) antigen specific immunoglobulins (antibodies).

- The genetic manipulations in the laboratory involving isolation and cloning of specific DNA fragments are collectively referred to as recombinant DNA technology. The technique involves the splicing of DNA by restriction endonucleases, preparation of chimeric DNA, followed by cloning for the production of large number of identical target DNA molecules.

- Polymerase chain reaction (PCR) is a novel test tube method for the amplification of a selected DNA fragment. It is specific, sensitive and rapid for the multiplication of DNA molecules.

- Southern blot, Northern blot and Western blot techniques are respectively, used for the specific identification of DNA, RNA and protein molecules.

- Restriction fragment length polymorphisms (RFLPs) are variations in the DNA structure that serve as DNA fingerprints for the identification of criminals and settling the disputes of parenthood.

- The practical applications of genetic engineering include production of proteins (insulin, interferon) in abundance, laboratory diagnosis of diseases (AIDS), molecular analysis of diseases (sickle-cell anemia), application in forensic medicine, gene therapy and study of evolution.

- Diabetes mellitus is a common metabolic disorder, characterized by insufficient or inefficient insulin.

- Insulin is a polypeptide hormone, secreted by the b–cells of pancreas. It has a profound influence on carbohydrate, fat and protein metabolisms. Insulin lowers blood glucose concentration (hypoglycemic effect).

- Glycagon, secreted by the α–cells of pancreas, in general opposes the actions of insulin. The net effect of glucagons is to increase blood glucose concentration (hyperglycemic effect).

- In a healthy person, the blood glucose level (fasting 70 – 100 mg/dl) is maintained by a well-coordinated hormonal action regulating the sources that contribute to glucose (gluconeogenesis, glyco-genolysis) and the utilization pathways (glycolysis, glycogenesis, lipogenesis). Insulin is hypoglycemic while other hormones (glucagons, epinephrine, thyroxine, glucocorticoids) are hyperglycemic.

- In hypoglycemia (blood glucose < 45 mg/dl), there is deprivation of glucose supply to brain resulting in symptoms such as headache, confusion, anxiety and seizures.

- Diabetes mellitus is broadly classified into 2 categories-insulin dependent diabetes mellitus (IDDM) and non-insulin dependent diabetes mellitus (NIDDM).

- The laboratory diagnosis of diabetes is frequently carried out by oral glucose tolerance test (GTT). As per WHO criteria a person is said to be suffering from diabetes if his/her fasting blood glucose exceeds 140 mg/dl and 2 hrs after oral glucose load goes beyond 200 mg/dl.

- Diabetes is associated with several metabolic derangements such as ketoacidosis and hypertriglyceridemia, besides hyperglycemia. The chronic complications of diabetes include atherosclerosis, retinopathy, nephropathy and neuropathy.

- Diet, exercise, drug and insulin are the options for diabetic control. It is estimated that about half of the new diabetic patients can be adequately controlled by diet and exercise.

- Estimation of glycated hemoglobin (HbA_1c), plasma fructosamine, micro albumins in urine and serum lipids serve as biochemical indices to monitor diabetic control.

- Cancer is characterized by uncontrolled cellular growth and development, leading to excessive proliferation and spread of cells. Cancer is the second largest killer disease (next to heart disease) in the developed world.

- Regulatory genes-namely oncogenes, antioncogenes and genes controlling cell death are involved in the development of cancer. Activation of oncogenes is a fundamental step in carcinogenesis. This may occur by insertion of viral DNA into host chromosome, translocation of chromosomes, gene amplification and point mutation.

- The products of activated oncogenes such as growth factors, growth factor receptors, GTP-binding proteins, and non-receptor tyrosine kinases have all been implicated in the development of cancer.

- Tumor markers of cancer include carcinoembryonic antigen (CEA), alpha-fetoprotein (AFP), cancer antigen-125 and prostate specific antigen (PSA). They are mainly useful to support diagnosis, monitor therapy and detect recurrence.

- There are several morphological and biochemical changes in the tumor cells, which distinguish them from the normal cells. The cancer cells are characterized by loss of contact inhibition, altered membrane transport, increased DNA and RNA synthesis, increased glycolysis, alteration in the structure of certain molecules.

- AIDS is a retroviral disease caused by human immunodeficiency virus (HIV). Immunosupression, secondary neoplasms and neurological manifestations characterize it. Transmission of HIV occurs by sexual contact (more in male homosexuals), parental inoculation (intravenous drug abusers) and from infected mothers to their newborns.

- HIV enters CD_4 T-lymphocytes where its genetic material RNA is transcribed into DNA by the enzyme reverse transcriptase. The viral DNA gets incorporated into the host genome ultimately leading to the multiplication of the virus and the destruction of CD_4 cells. This is the root cause of immunosupression leading to opportunistic infections in AIDS.

- The natural course of AIDS has 3 distinct phases-acute, chronic and crisis. A patient with lower than 200 CD_4 T-lymphocytes 1 ml is considered to have developed AIDS. The sensitive laboratory tests for AIDS detection are ELISA, Western blot technique and recently, PCR.

- There is no cure for AIDS. The patients generally die within 5-10 years after HIV infection. Administrations of drugs (zidovudine and didanosine), however, prolong the life of AIDS patients. These drugs inhibit the viral enzyme reverse transcriptase and halt the multiplication of the virus.

- The attempts to produce vaccine for AIDS have been unsuccessful due to the variations in the genome (and therefore, the protein products) of the HIV.

- The general principles of organic chemistry provide strong foundations in understanding biochemistry, despite the fact that the latter exclusively deals with living system.

- Biomolecules possess certain functional groups (aldehyde, keto, alcohol, acid, amino), which are the reaction centers.

- Several homocyclic and heterocyclic ring structures are commonly encountered in biochemistry. These include phenyl ring, purine, pyrimidine and thiophene.

- Isomerism refers to the existence of different structures (isomers) with the same molecular formula. It is of two types—structural isomerism and stereoisomerism.

- Geometrical isomerism is due to the restriction of freedom of rotation of the groups around carbon-carbon double bond.

- Optical isomerism is due to the characteristic property of certain compounds to rotate the plane of polarized light, which is attributed to the asymmetric (chiral) carbon.

- The basic principles of chemistry and physics are important to understand the physico-chemical aspects of life.

- Water is the solvent of life. Its properties have profound biological significance to maintain aqueous environment and sustain life.

- An acid is proton (H^+) donor while a base is proton acceptor. PH is defined as the negative logarithm of H^+ ion concentration. Buffers are solutions, which resist change in pH by the addition of small amount of acids or bases.

- Colloidal state is a heterogeneous two-phase system, characterized by the particle size of 1 to 10 mm. Example of biological colloids include blood, milk and cerebrospinal fluid.

- Diffusion is a free movement of solute molecules from a higher concentration to a lower concentration. Exchange of gases in the lungs and tissues occurs by diffusion.

- Osmosis refers to the movement of solvent molecules through a semi-permeable membrane. It is a collective property that depends on the number of particles and not on their nature.

- In Donnan membrane equilibrium, the presence of non-diffusible ions influences the concentration of diffusible ions across the membrane. This causes difference in the distribution of ions in the biological fluids, membrane hydrolysis and difference in the osmotic pressure.

- Viscosity is the internal resistance offered by a liquid to its flow. Surface tension refers to the force with which the molecules on the surface of a liquid are held together.

- Isotopes are the atoms with the same atomic number but different atomic weights. Radioactive isotopes are of immense importance in biochemical research, particularly for elucidating metabolic reactions.

- Liquid scintillation counter is the most commonly used equipment in the laboratory to measure the radioactivity of isotopes.

- The foundations for the existing knowledge of biochemistry are derived from the laboratory tools of biochemistry. These include chromatography, electrophoresis, photometry, ultracentrifugation, radioimmunoassay, recombinant DNA technology, ELISA, use of radioisotopes and polymerase chain reaction (PCR).

- Chromatography primarily deals with the separation of closely related compounds from a mixture, e.g., amino acids, lipids, carbohydrates, vitamins, and drugs. The separation is based on the physico-chemical principles such as partition, adsorption, ion exchange and affinity.

- Ion-exchange chromatography separates molecules on the basis of their ionic charges. The principle of separation is based on the molecular size in gel-filtration chromatography.

- Electrophoresis, the movement of charged particles in an electric field, is frequently employed in the laboratory as a separation technique for biological molecules, e.g., proteins, lipoproteins, and immunoglobulins.

- Colorimeter and spectrophotometer are the instruments used for the quantitative estimation of specific compounds of interest in the biological samples. Their working is based on Beer-Lambert law.

- Fluorimetry works on the principle of measuring fluorescence. For flame photometer, it is the emission light that is detected.

- Ultracentrifuge is useful for the isolation of subcellular particles, proteins and nucleic acids. In addition, this equipment also helps in the determination of molecular weight of macromolecules.

- The development of radioimmunoassay (RIA) has revolutionized the estimation of several compounds in biological fluids in exceedingly low concentration (nanogram or picogram), e.g., hormones, drugs.

- Enzymes-linked immunosorbant assay (ELISA) is a simple non-isotopic immunoassay, which is as sensitive as or even more sensitive than RIA.

- Hybridoma technology deals with the unlimited production of antibodies with defined specificities (monoclonal antibodies).

10

CLINICAL BIOCHEMICAL
SHORT EXPLANATIONS

- The most common organic compounds of living systems are carbohydrates, lipids, proteins, nucleic acids and vitamins.
- One type of optical isomers (D or L) is commonly encountered in living cells. Amino acids are of L-type, while carbohydrates are of D-type.
- The aqueous environment of water maintains the structures of Biomolecules.
- The biological system has several buffers to resist alterations in pH, e.g., bicarbonate buffer, phosphate buffer, protein buffers.
- Fat digestion and absorption are facilitated through the formation of emulsions by the bile salts.
- Glucose is converted to other carbohydrates. These include glycogen for storage, ribose for nucleic acid synthesis and galactose for lactose formation.
- Fructose is abundantly found in the serum, which is utilized by the sperms for energy.
- Several diseases are associated with carbohydrates, e.g., diabetes mellitus, glycogen storage diseases, galactosemia.
- Insulin a polymer of fructose is used to assess renal function by measuring glomerular filtration rate (GFR).
- The non-digestible carbohydrate cellulose plays a significant role in human nutrition. These include decreasing the intestinal absorption of glucose and cholesterol and increasing bulk of feces to avoid constipation.
- The mucopolysaccharide hyaluronic acid serves as a lubricant and shock absorbent in joints.
- The enzyme hyaluronidase of semen degrades the gel (contains hyaluronic acid) around the ovum. This allows effective penetration of sperm into the ovum.
- The mucopolysaccharide heparin is an anticoagulant (prevents blood clotting).

- The survival of Antarctic fish below −2°C is attributed to the antifreeze glycoproteins.

- Streptomycin is a glycoside employed in the treatment of tuberculosis.

- Lipids are important to the body as constituents of membranes, source of fat soluble (A, D, E and K) vitamins and metabolic regulations (steroid hormones and prostaglandins).

- Triacylglycerols (fats) primarily stored in the adipose tissue are concentrated fuel reserves of the body. Fats found in the subcutaneous tissue and around certain organs serve as thermal insulators.

- The unsaturated fatty acids—linoleic and linolenic acid are essential to human, the deficiency of which causes phrynoderma or toad skin.

- The cyclic fatty acid, namely chaulmoogric acid is employed in the treatment of leprosy.

- Fats and oils on exposure to air, moisture, bacteria etc. undergo rancidity (deterioration). This can be prevented by the addition of certain antioxidants (vitamin E, hydroquinone, gallic acid).

- In food preservation, antioxidants namely propyl gallate, butylated hydroanisole and butylated hydroxyl toluene are commonly used.

- The phospholipid-dipalmitoyl lecithin-prevents the adherence of inner surface of the lungs, the absence of which is associated with respiratory distress syndrome in infants.

- Cephalins participate in blood clotting.

- The action of certain hormones is mediated through phosphatidylinositol.

- Phospholipids are important for the synthesis and transport of lipoproteins and reserve transport of cholesterol.

- Cholesterol is essential for the synthesis of bile acids, hormones (sex and cortical) and vitamin D.

- Lipoproteins occur in the membrane structure, besides serving as a means of transport vehicles for lipids.

- Lipids are associated with the disorders—obesity and atherosclerosis.

- Proteins are the most abundant organic molecules of life. They perform static (structural) and dynamic functions in the living cells.

- The dynamic functions of proteins are highly derived field such as enzymes, hormones, clotting factors, immunoglobulins, storage proteins and membrane receptors.

- Half of the amino acids (about 10) that occur in proteins have to be consumed by humans in the diet, hence they are essential.

- A protein is said to be complete (or first class) protein if all the essential amino acids are present in the required proportion by the human body, e.g., egg albumin.

- Cooking results in protein denaturation exposing more peptide bonds for easy digestion.

- Collagen is the most abundant protein in mammals. It is rich in dyhroxyproline and hydroxylysine.

- Several biological important peptides are known in the living organism. These include glutathione for the maintenance of RBC structure and integrity; oxytocin that causes uterus contraction; vasopressin that stimulates retention of water by kidney; enkephalins that inhibit the sense of pain in the brain.

- Antibodies such as actinomycin, gramicidin, bacitracin and tyrocidin are peptide in nature.

- γ-Carboxyglutamic acid is an amino acid derivative found in certain plasma proteins involved in blood clotting.

- Several non-protein amino acids of biological importance are known. These include ornithine, citrulline and arginosuccinic acid (intermediates of urea synthesis), thyroxin and triiodothyroxine (hormones), S-adenosyl-methionine (methyl donor) and β–alanine (a component of coenzyme A).

- The protein-free filtrate of blood, required for biochemical investigations (e.g., urea, sugar) can be obtained by using protein-precipitating agents such as phosphotungstic acid and trichloro acetic acid.

- Heat coagulation test is most commonly employed to detect the presence of albumin in urine.

- DNA is the reserve bank of genetic information, ultimately responsible for the chemical basis of life and heredity.

- DNA is organized into genes, the fundamental units of genetic information. Genes control protein biosynthesis through the mediation of RNA.

- It is estimated that the 23 pairs of human chromosomes contain about 100,000 genes. The total contour length of the entire DNA in a single human cell is about 2 meters. An adult human body has 10^{14} cells. Thus the total length of DNA in the human body is about 2×10^{10} km, i.e., 20 billion Km. This is much higher than the distance between the earth and the sun (1.5×10^8 Km).

- Nucleic acids are the polymers of nucleotides. Certain nucleotides serve B-complex vitamin coenzymes (FAD, NAD^+, CoA), carriers of high-energy intermediates (UDP-glucose, S-adenosylmethionine) and second messengers of hormonal action (cAMP, cGMP).

- Uric acid is a purine and the end product of purine metabolism, which has been implicated in the disorder gout.

- Certain purine bases from plants such as caffeine (of coffee), theophylline (of tea) and theobromine (of cocoa) are of pharmacological interest.

- Synthetic analogs of bases (5-fluorouracil, 6-mercaptopurine, 6-azauridine) are used to inhibit the growth of cancer cells.

- The existence of life is unimaginable without the presence of enzymes-the biocatalysts.

- Majority of the coenzymes (TPP, NAD+, FAD, CoA) are derived from B-complex vitamins in which form the latter exert their biochemical functions.

- Competitive inhibitors of certain enzymes are of great biological significance. Albpurinol, employed in the treatment of gout, inhibits xanthine oxidase to reduce the formation of uric acid. The other competitive inhibitors include amino pterin used in the treatment of cancers, sulphanil amide as antibactericidal agent and dicumarol as an anticoagulant.

- The nerve gas (diisopropyl fluorophosphates), first developed by Germans during Second World War, inhibits acetylcholine esterase, the enzyme essential for nerve conduction and paralyses the vital body functions. Many organophosphorus insecticides (e.g., melathion) also block the activity of acetylcholine esterase.

- Penicillin antibiotics irreversibly inhibit serine-containing enzymes of bacterial cell wall synthesis.

- In the living system, the regulation of enzyme activities occurs through allosteric inhibition, activation of latent enzymes, compartmentation of metabolic pathways, control of enzyme synthesis and degradation.

- Feedback (or end product) inhibition is a specialized form of allosteric inhibition that controls several metabolic pathways, e.g., CTP inhibits aspartate transcarbamoylase; cholesterol inhibits HMG CoA reductase. The end product inhibition is utmost important to cellular economy since a compound is synthesized only when required.

- Certain RNA molecules (ribozymes) function as non-protein enzymes. It is believed that ribozymes were functioning as biocatalysts before the occurrence of protein enzymes during evolution.

- Certain enzymes are utilized as therapeutic agents. Streptokinase in used to dissolve blood clots in circulation while asparaginase is employed in the treatment of leukemias.

- Determination of serum enzyme activities is of great importance for the diagnosis of several diseases.

- Lowered body temperature (hypothermia) is accompanied by a decrease in enzyme activities. This principle is exploited to reduce metabolic demand during open-heart surgery or transportation of organs for transplantation surgery.

- It is believed that during the course of evolution, the ability to synthesize vitamins was lost by the higher organisms; hence they should be supplied through the diet.

- For humans the normal intestinal bacterial synthesis of vitamin K and biotin is almost sufficient to meet the body requirements.

- Administration of antibiotics often destroys the vitamin-synthesizing bacteria in the gut, hence additional supplementation of vitamins is recommended during antibiotic therapy.

- Vitamin A deficiency causes night blindness; vitamin D deficiency rickets (in children) or osteomalacia (in adults); vitamin E deficiency minor neurological symptoms; vitamin K deficiency bleeding.

- Fat-soluble vitamins are not readily excreted in urine, hence excess consumption leads to their accumulation and toxic effects.

- Vitamin C deficiency causes scurvy. The manifestations of scurvy are related to the impairment in the synthesis of collagen and/or the antioxidant property of vitamin C.

- Mega doses of vitamin C are used in common cold, wound healing, trauma etc.

- β-Carotene, vitamin E and ascorbic acid serve as antioxidants and reduce the risk of heart attacks and cancers.

- Water-soluble vitamins form coenzymes that participate in variety of biochemical reactions, most of which are related to either energy production or hematopoiesis.

- Distinct deficiency conditions of certain B-complex vitamins are known.

Thiamine	Beri-beri
Riboflavin	Cheilosis, glossitis
Niacin	Pellagra
Pyridoxine	Peripheral neuropathy
Folic acid	Macrocytic anemia
Cobalamin	Pernicious anemia

- B-complex vitamin deficiencies are usually multiple rather than individual with over lapping symptoms.

- A combined therapy of vitamin B_{12} and folic acid is commonly employed to treat the patients of megaloblastic anemias.

- Mega doses of niacin are useful in the treatment of hyper lipidemia.

- Long-term use of isoniazide for the treatment of tuberculosis causes B_6 deficiency.

- High consumption of raw eggs (contain avidin) may lead to biotin deficiency.

- Sulfonamides serve as antibacterial drugs by inhibiting the incorporation of PABA to produce folic acid.

- Aminopterin and amethopterin, the structural analogues of folic acid are employed in the treatment of cancers.

- Cooking of food significantly improves the digestibility by enzymes.

  lactose intolerance due to a defect in the enzyme lactase (β-galactosidase) is very common. The treatment advocated is severe restriction of lactose (milk and milk products) in the diet.

- Flatulence occurring after ingestion of certain non-digestible oligosaccharides is characterized by increased intestinal motility, cramps and irritability.

- Direct intestinal absorption of proteins and polypeptides is observed in the infants, immediately after birth. This is important for the transfer of maternal immunoglobins (via-breast-feeding to the offspring).

- In some adults, macromolecular (protein) absorption by intestine is responsible for antibody formation, often causing food allergy.

- Hartnup's disease is characterized by an important in the absorption of neutral amino acids (particularly tryptophan) by intestinal and renal epithelial cells.

- Emulsification of lipids is essential for their effective digestion since lipases can act only on the surface of lipid droplets.

- Bile salts are the most efficient biological emulsifying agents.

- Steatorrhea, characterized by the loss of lipids in feces is commonly associated with impaired pancreatic function and biliary obstruction. Peptic ulcers occur due to the auto digestion of mucosa by gastric secretions (pepsin and HCl).

- Acute pancreatitis is caused by auto digestion of pancreas while chronic pancreatitis is associated with excessive consumption of alcohol.

- Albumin, the most abundant plasma protein, is involved in osmotic function, transport of several compounds (fatty acids, steroid hormones) besides the buffering action.

- α_1-Antitrypsin deficiency has been implicated in emphysema (abnormal distension of lungs by air), which is more commonly associated with heavy smoking.

- Haptoglobin prevents the possible loss of free hemoglobin from the plasma through the kidneys by forming haptoglobin-hemoglobin complex.

- Man and other animals have evolved a defense system (immunity) to protect themselves against the invasion of foreign substances such as viruses, bacteria or proteins. Immunoglobulins (antibodies) a specialized group of plasma globular proteins, are actively involved in immunity.

- IgG and IgM are primarily concerned with humoral immunity while IgE is associated with allergic reactions.

- Multiple myeloma, a plasma cell cancer disease of bone marrow, is characterized by over production of abnormal immunoglobulins (mostly IgG). Laboratory diagnosis of multiple myeloma can be made by the presence of a distinct M band on plasma/serum electrophoresis.

- Blood clotting or coagulation is the body's major defense mechanism against blood loss. Defense in clotting factors cause coagulation abnormalities such as hemophilia A (deficiency of factor VIII) and Christmas disease (deficiency of factor IX).

- Anticoagulants inhibit blood clotting. These include heparin, oxalate, fluoride, EDTA and citrate.

- Hemoglobin is primarily responsible for the delivery of O_2 from lungs to tissue and the transport of CO_2 from tissue to lungs.

- Increased erythrocyte 2,3-BPG levels in anemia and chronic hypoxia facilitate the release of more O_2 from the oxyhemoglobin to the tissues.

- Storage of blood causes a decrease in the concentration of 2,3-BPG. This can be prevented by the addition of ionosine.

- Hemoglobin (Fe^{++}) on oxidation by H_2O_2, free radicals or drugs, forms methemoglobin (Fe^{+++}), which cannot transport O_2.

- Carboxyhemoglobin is produced when carbon monoxide, an industrial pollutant, binds to hemoglobin. The clinical manifestations of CO toxicity (> 20% COHb) include headache, nausea, breathlessness and vomiting.

- Sickle cell hemoglobin (Hbs) causes hemolytic anemia, increased susceptibility to infection and premature death, However, Hbs offers protection against malaria.

- Thalassemias are hemolytic disorders caused by impairedment/ imbalance in the synthesis of globin chains of Hb. These include α-thalassemia trait, hydrops fetalis and β-thalassemias.

- Abnormalities in heme synthesis cause porphytias, which may be erythropoietic (enzyme defect in RBC) or hepatic (enzyme defect in liver). Porphyries are associated with elevated excretion of porphyries, neuro psychiatric disturbances and cardiovascular abnormalities.

- Jaundice is caused by elevated serum bilirubin (normal < 0.8 mg/dl) elevated and is characterized by yellow coloration of white of the eyes and skin.

- The most important function of food is to supply energy to the living cells. This is finally achieved through biological oxidation.

- The supply of O_2 is very essential for the survival of life (exception- anaerobic bacteria).

- ATP, the energy currency of the cell, acts as a link between the catabolism and anabolism in the living system. The major production of body's ATP occurs in the mitochondria through oxidative phosphorylation coupled with respiration.

- Respiration chain or electron transport chain (ETC) is blocked by site specific inhibitors such as rotenone, amytal, antimycin A, BAL, carbon monoxide and cyanide.

- Uncoupling of respiration from oxidative phosphorylation under natural conditions assumes biological significance. The brown adipose tissue, rich in electron carriers, brings about oxidation uncoupled from phosphorylation.

- Inherited disorders of oxidative phosphorylation caused by the mutations in mitochondrial DNA have been identified, e.g., Leber's hereditary optic neuropathy.

- The partially reduced species of oxygen (notably superoxide) are highly reactive and can damage DNA, unsaturated lipids and proteins. They have also been implicated in cancer, ageing and inflammation. The living cells, however, possess certain defense mechanism (particularly superoxide dismutase) to combat the adverse effects of O_2 radicals.

- The superoxide liberated during phagocytosis is believed to be involved in killing the bacteria.

- The basic metabolic pathways in most organisms are essentially identical.

- The metabolic reactions or pathways do not occur in isolation. They are interdependent and integrated.

- The inborn errors of metabolism in higher organisms and the genetic manipulations in the microorganisms have largely contributed to our understanding of metabolisms.

- Glycolysis is an important source of energy supply for brain, retina, skin and renal medulla.

- The crucial significance of glycolysis is its ability to generate ATP in the absence of oxygen.

- Skeletal muscle, during strenuous exercise, requires the occurrence of uninterrupted glycolysis. This is due to the limited supply of oxygen.

- The cardiac muscle cannot survive for long in the absence of oxygen since it is not well adapted for glycolysis under anaerobic conditions.

- Glycolysis erythrocytes are associated with 2,3-bisphophoglycerate (2, 3-BPG) production. In the presence of 2, 3-BPG, oxyhemoglobin unloads more oxygen to the tissues.

- The occurrence of glycolysis is very much elevated in rapidly growing cancer cells.

- In alcoholics with thiamine deficiency, more pyruvate is diverted to lactate formation, resulting in lactic acidsosis.

- Lactic acidosis is also observed in patients with deficiency of the enzyme pyruvate dehydrogenase.

- Citric acid cycle is the final common oxidative pathway for carbohydrates, fats and amino acids. It utilizes (in directly) about 2/3 of the total oxygen consumed by the body and generates about 2/3 of the total energy (ATP).

- Kerbs cycle is unique as it integrates-either directly or indirectly almost all the metabolisms in the body. This pathway is involved in gluconeogesis, lipogenesis, synthesis of heme and amino acids, transamination etc.

- Unlike the other metabolic pathways/cycles, very few genetic abnormalities of Krebs cycle are known. This may be due to the vital importance of this metabolic cycle for the survival of life.

- A continuous presence of glucose-supplied through diet or synthesized in the body (gluconeogenesis) is essential for the survival of the organism.

- Human brain consumes about 120 g of glucose per day out of the 160 g needed by the body. Insufficient supply of glucose to brain may lead to coma and death.

- Liver glycogen serves as an immediate source for maintaining blood glucose levels, particularly between the meals. The glycogen stress in the liver gets depleted after 12–18 hours of fasting.

- Muscle glycogen is primarily concerned with the supply of hexoses that undergo glycolysis to provide energy during muscle contraction.

- In ruminants a fatty acid-propionate-formed during the course of carbohydrate digestion is a good precursor for gluconeogenesis in these species.

- Glycogen storage diseases-characterized by deposition normal or abnormal type of glycogen in one or more tissues-result in muscular weakness or even death.

- The occurrence of HMP shunt (NADPH production) in the RBC is necessary to maintain the integrity of erythrocyte membrane and to prevent the accumulation of methemoglbin.

- Deficiency of glucose 6-phosphate dehydrogenase results in hemolysis of RBC, causing hemolytic anemia. The subjects of G6PD deficiency are, however, resistant to malaria.

- Uronic acid pathway is concerned with the production of glucuronic acid (involved in detoxification), pentoses and vitamin C. Man is incapable of synthesizing vitamin C due to the absence of a single enzyme L-gulonolactone oxidase.

- The conversion of glucose to fructose is impaired in diabetes mellitus, causing accumulation of sorbitol. This compound has been implicated in the development of cataract, nephropathy, and peripheral neuropathy.

- Severe cases of galctosemia are associated with the development of cataract, believed to be due to the accumulation of galactitol.

- An adult human body contains about 10 – 11 Kg of fat reserve corresponding to about 100, 000 Cal. This can meet the energy requirements for several weeks of food deprivation in man.

- The sudden infant death syndrome (SIDS) an unexpected overnight death of healthy infants is attributed to a blockade in β–oxidation of fatty acids caused by a deficiency of medium chain acyl CoA dehyrogenase (MCAD).

- Jamaican vomiting sickness is due to consumption of unripe ackee fruit containing hypoglycin, A which blocks β–oxidation.

- Methylmalonic academia occurs either due to a deficiency of the vitamin B_{12} or a defect in an enzyme methyl malonyl CoA mutase. This disorder retards growth and damages central nervous system.

- Zellweger syndrome is caused by absence of peroxisomes in tissue; as a result, the long chain fatty acids cannot be oxidized.

- Refsum's disease is due to a defect in oxidation of fatty acids. The patients are advised not to consume diets containing chlorophyll.

- Ketosis is commonly associated with uncontrolled diabetes mellitus and starvation. Diabetes ketoacidosis is dangerous may result in coma or even death. Starvation, however, is not accompanied by ketoacidosis.

- Insulin promotes fatty acid synthesis by stimulating the conversion of pyruvate to acetyl CoA.

- The lack of the ability of the organisms to introduce double bonds in fatty acids beyond C_9 and C_{10} makes linoleic and linolenic acids essential to mammals.

- Niemann-Pick disease, caused by a defect in the enzyme sphingo-myelinase, results in the accumulation of sphingomyelins in liver and spleen.

- About a dozen glycolipid storage diseases are known. These include Gaucher's disease and Krabbe's disease.

- Hyper cholesterolemia is associated with atherosclerosis and coronary diseases. Consumption of polyunsaturated fatty acids and fiber decreases cholesterol in circulation.

- Drugs such as lovastatin, cholestyramine, compactin and clofibrate reduce plasma cholesterol.

- Cholelithiasis a cholesterol gall stone disease is caused by a defect in the absorption of bile salts from the intestine or biliary tract obstruction.

- High-density lipoproteins in association with lecithin-cholesterol acyltransferase (LCAT) are responsible for the transport and elimination of cholesterol from the body.

- Hyper lipoproteinemias are a group of disorders caused by the elevation of one or more of plasma lipoprotein fractions.

- Excessive accumulation of triacylglycerols causes fatty liver, which can be prevented by the consumption of lipoptropic factors (choline, betaine, methionine).

- Obesity is an abnormal increase in body weight due to excessive fat deposition (> 25%). Over eating, lack of exercise and genetic predisposition play a significant role in the development of obesity.

- Some individuals with active brown adipose tissue do not become obese despite over eating, since whatever they eat is liberated as heat due to uncoupling of oxidation and phosphorylation in the mitochondria.

- A protein namely leptin, produced by the adipose tissue, has been identified (1994) in mice. Injection of leptin to obese mice caused reduction in body fat, increased metabolic rate and increased insulin concentration, besides reduced food intake. Leptin has also been detected in humans.

- Anorexia nervosa is a psychiatric disorder associated with total loss of appetite mostly found in females in the age group 10-30 years.

- Atherosclerosis is characterized by hardening of arteries due to the accumulation of lipids and other compounds. The probable causes of atherosclerosis include hyper lipoproteinemias, diabetes mellitus, obesity, high consumption of saturated fat lack of exercise and stress.

- Atherosclerosis and coronary heart disease are directly correlated with plasma cholesterol and LDL, inversely with HDL. Elevation of plasma lipoprotein suggests increased risk of CHD.

- Alcoholism is associated with fatty liver, hyperlipidemia and atherosclerosis.

- About 300–400 g of protein per day is constantly degraded and synthesized in the human body.

- The amino acids are mainly utilized for protein biosynthesis, production of specialized products (creatine, porphyrin, amines, purines, pyrimidines) and generation of energy.

- Glutamate is the collection center for the amino groups in the biological system while glutamine is the storehouse of NH_3. Free NH_3 can be liberated predominantly from glutamate.

- Ammonia accumulation in blood is toxic to brain causing slurring of speech, blurring of vision, tremors and even death. Mammals convert NH_3 to urea, a non-toxic excretory product. Metabolic defects in urea cycle enzymes results in hyper ammonemia.

- Dietary consumption of a protein rich meal increases the level of N-acetylglutamate in liver, which enhances urea production.

- Primary hyper oxaluria a metabolic disorder due to a defect in the enzyme glycine transaminase is characterized by elevated urinary oxalate and the formation of oxalate stones.

- Blood urea estimation is commonly used to assess renal function. Elevation of blood urea level (normal 10 – 40 mg/dl) is associated with several disorders which may be prerenal (diabetic coma), renal (acute glomerulonephritis) and post-renal (tumors or stones in the urinary tract).

- Estimation of serum creatinine (normal > 1 mg/dl) is considered to be a more reliable indicator for the evaluation of kidney function.

- Melanin-the pigment of skin, hair and eyes is produced from tyrosine. Lack of melanin synthesis (mostly due to a deficiency of tyrosinase) causes albinism.

- Parkinson's disease a common disorder of the elderly is linked with decreased synthesis of dopamine. It is characterized by muscular rigidity, tremors, and lethargy.

- Phenylketonuria, due to a defect in the enzyme phenylalanine hydroxylase is characterized by failure of growth, seizures and mental retardation (Low IQ).

- Alkaptonuria causes the accumulation of homogentisate, which undergoes oxidation followed by polymerization to produce the pigment alkapton. Deposition of alkapton in tissues (connective tissue, bones) causes ochronosis, which is associated with arthritis.

- Serotonin an excitatory neurotransmitter is synthesized from tryptophan. Psychin stimulant drugs (isoniazide) elevate serotonin levels while depressant drugs (LSD) decrease.

- Malignant carcinoid syndrome, a tumor of argentaffin cells of gastro intestinal tract is characterized by tremendously increased production of serotonin. The elevated levels of 5-hydroxyindoleacetate in urine can diagnose this disorder.

- Melatonin produced from serotonin, is involved in circadian rhythms or diurnal variations, i.e., maintenance of body's biological clock.

- Homocysteine has been implicated as a risk factor in the onset of coronary heart diseases.

- Hisitidine loading test characterized by elevated excretion of N-formiminoglutamate (FIGLU) is commonly employed to assess the deficiency of the vitamin folic acid.

- Nitric oxide synthesized from arginine is involved in several biological functions vasodilatation, platelet aggregation, neurotransmission, and bacterial action.

- g-Amino butyric acid (GABA), produced from glutamate is an inhibitory neurotransmitter low level of GABA result in convulsions.

- The carbon skeleton of amino acids may be converted to glucose (glycogenic) or fat (ketogenic), besides being responsible for the synthesis of non-essential amino acids

- Polyamines (spermine, putrescine) are involved in the synthesis of DNA, RNA and proteins and thus are essential for cell growth and differentiation.

- Biochemists for their convenience learn body chemical processes in terms of individual metabolic reactions and pathways, although thousands of reactions simultaneously occur in a living cell.

- The metabolic pathways in various tissues and organs are well coordinated to meet the demands of the body.

- Liver is appropriately regarded as the body's central metabolic clearinghouse while adipose tissues constitute the energy (fat) storehouse.

- Brain is a vital metabolic organ that consumes about 20% of body's oxygen, although it constitutes only 2% of body weight.

- The metabolism in starvation is recognized to meet the body's changed demands and metabolic compulsions.

- Under normal circumstances, glucose is the only fuel source to brain. However, during starvation, the brain slowly gets adapted to use ketone bodies for energy needs.

- Folic acid is essential for the synthesis of purine nucleotides. Folic acid analogs (methotrexate) are employed to control cancer.

- The salvage pathway, involving the direct conversion of purines to corresponding nucleotides is important in tissues-brain and erythrocytes.

- Gout is the disorder associated with the overproduction of uric acid, the end product of purine metabolism. Albpurinol is the drug of choice for the treatment of gout.

- Lesch-Nyhan syndrome is caused by a defect in the enzyme hypoxanthine-guanine phosphoribosyl transferase. The patients have an irresistible urge to bite their fingers and lips.

- A defect in the enzyme adenosine deaminase (ADA) results in severe combined immunodeficiency (SCID) involving both T-cell and B-cell dysfunction. A girl suffering from SCID was cured by transferring ADA gene (in 1990) and that was the first attempt for gene therapy in modern medicine.

- Orotic aciduria a metabolic defect in pyrimidine biosynthesis is characterized by anemia and retarded growth, besides the excretion of orotic acid in urine.

- A few micrograms (10 g) of DNA in a fetal cell stores the genetic information that will determine the differentiation and every function of an adult animal. This is the marvel of molecular biology.

- An error-free synthesis of DNA (replication) is essential for the very existence of the organism. This is achieved by a proof reading activity of DNA polymerase.

- The use of naked DNA (DNA that is freed from all natural proteins) as vaccine is gaining importance in recent years. It appears that DNA vaccines stimulate hormonal as well as cell mediated immune responses.

- DNA is constantly subjected to damage by environment insults and replication errors. Fortunately, the cells posses an excellent repairing machinery to undo the damage done to DNA.

- Xeroderma pigmentation characterized by hyper pigmentation and skin cancers is due to a defect in the DNA repair caused by UV rays.

- Inhibitors of RNA synthesis (transcription) are employed as therapeutic agents. Thus, actinomycin D was the first antibiotic used in the treatment of tumors. Rifampin is used to treat tuberculosis and leprosy.

- Retroviruses (RNA is the genetic material) are oncogenic can cause cancer in animals.

- Several antibiotics are known to inhibit bacterial protein synthesis. These include streptomycin, tetracycline, puromycin and erythromycin.

- The mitochondrial DNA (mtDNA) is inherited from the mother since the sperm cell mitochondria do not enter the ovum during fertilization.

- Leber's hereditary optic neuropathy is caused by mutation in mtDNA in males. The victims become blind due to loss of central vision.

- Mutations results in a permanent change in DNA structure, which have been implicated in the etiopathogenesis of cancer.

- Certain anti-cancer agents (anthracyline, aminoacridine, camptothecin) act on the enzymes, topoisomerases and block the rejoining of DNA strands, finally leading to cell death.

- Genetic engineering to medical and agricultural sciences that has immensely benefited mankind.

- An abundant production of DNA in a test tube has been successfully achieved by polymerase chain reaction.

- DNA probes are now available for the detection of certain genetic disorders.

- RFLPs serve as DNA fingerprints for the identification (by Southern blot technique) of criminals or in settling the disputes of parenthood.

- The human genome contains about 100, 000 genes. Through the application of genetic engineering techniques, it is expected that the entire sequence of human genome will be known soon.

- Serum calcium level is increased (normal 9–111 mg/dl) in hyper-parathyroidism. This condition is also associated with elevated urinary excretion of Ca and P, often leading to stone formation.

- Tetany caused by a drastic reduction in serum Ca is characterized by neuromuscular irritability and convulsions.

- Rickets is due to defective calcification of bones. This may be caused by deficiency of Ca and P or vitamin D or both.

- Osteoporosis is the bone disorder of the elderly characterized by demineralization resulting in a progressive loss of bone mass. It is the major cause of bone fractures and disability in the old people.

- Decrease levels of serum Na^+ (hyponatremia) is observed in diarrhea and vomiting, besides Addison's disease, while increase serum Na^+ (hypernatremia) is found in Cushing's syndrome.

- Iron deficiency anemia is the most prevalent nutritional disorder world over. It is most commonly observed in pregnant and lactating women.

- Wilson's disease is due to an abnormal copper metabolism. It is characterized by abnormal deposition of copper in liver and brain, besides the low levels of plasma copper and ceruloplasmin.

- Endemic goiter, due to dietary iodine deficiency is very common. Consumption of iodized salt is advocated to overcome this problem.

- Fluorosis is caused by an excessive intake of fluoride. The manifestations include mottling of enamel and discoloration of teeth. In the advanced stages, hyper calcification of limb bones and ligaments of spine get calcified, ultimately crippling the individual.

- Existence of life is unimaginable in the absence of water.

- Kidneys play predominant role in the regulation of water, electrolyte and acid-base balance.

- Electrolyte and water balance regulation occurs through the involvement of hormones aldosterone, ADH and rennin-angiotensin.

- Low blood pressure; sunken eyeballs, lethargy, confusion and coma characterize severe dehydration.

- Sodium is the principal extracellular cation while potassium is intracellular. The maintenance of the differential concentration of these electrolytes is essential for the survival of life, which is brought about by the Na^+-K^+ pump.

- The body metabolism is accompanied by the production of acids such as carbonic acid, sulfuric acid, phosphoric acid etc.

- Vegetarian diet has an alkalizing effect on the body. This is attributed to the formation of organic acids such as sodium lactate, which can deplete H^+ ions by combining with them.

- Blood buffers, respiratory and renal mechanisms, maintain the blood pH.

- Carbon dioxide is the central molecule of acid-base regulation.

- Disturbances in acid-base regulation result in acidosis (decreased blood pH) or alkalosis (raised blood pH).

- Uncontrolled diabetes mellitus is associated with metabolic acidosis, commonly referred to as ketoacidosis (due to the overproduction of ketone bodies).

- Hypothalamus of the brain is the master coordinator of hormonal action. It liberates certain releasing factors or hormones, which stimulate or inhibit the release of corresponding tropic hormones from the anterior pituitary which, in turn act on the target endocrine organs.

- Growth hormone deficiency causes dwarfism while its excessive production results in gigantism (in children) or acromegaly (in adults).

- Identification of HCG in urine is employed for the early detection of pregnancy.

- Cushing syndrome is due to overproduction of ACTH that results in the increased synthesis of adrenocorticosteroids. The symptoms of this syndrome include hypertension, edema and negative nitrogen balance.

- Endorphins and enkephalins are the natural painkillers in the brain. It is believed that the pain relief through acupuncture and placebos is mediated through these compounds.

- Deficiency of ADH causes diabetes insipidus, a disorder characterized by excretion of large volumes of dilute urine (polyuria).

- Thyroid hormones directly influence Na^+-K^+ ATP pump which consumes a major share cellular ATP. Obesity in some individuals is attributed to decreased energy utilization (heat production) due to diminished Na^+-K^+ ATPase activity.

- Catecholamines are produced in response to fight, fright and flight. The ultimate goal of catecholamine function is to mobilize energy resources and prepare the individual to meet emergencies such as shock, cold, fatigue, anger etc.

- Pheochromocytomas are the tumors of adrenal medulla, characterized by excessive production of epinephrine and norepinephrine, associated with severe hypertension.

- Sex hormones are primarily responsible for growth, development, maintenance and regulation of reproductive system.

- The low incidence of atherosclerosis and coronary heart diseases in the women during reproductive age is due to estrogens.

- The impairment in the function of any organ in the body wills adversely influences the health of the organism. Organ function tests are the laboratory tools to biochemically evaluate the working of a given organ.

- Acute viral hepatitis is associated with elevated alanine transaminase (predominantly) aspartate transaminase and bilirubin.

- Increase in serum γ–glutamyl transpeptidase is observed in biliary obstruction and alcoholism.

- A combination of laboratory investigations instead of a single one is commonly employed in assessing function. Kidney function can be accurately assessed by clearance tests, measuring glomerular filtration rate. A reduction in clearance reflects renal damage.

- Zollinger-Ellison syndrome, a tumor of gastrin secreting cells of the pancreas is associated with increased gastric HCl production.

- Most of the information on human nutrition is based on the research carried out in experimental animals.

- The body at total rest (physical and mental) requires energy to meet the basal requirements such as working of heart, conduction of nerve impulse, membrane transport etc.

- Carbohydrates are the most abundant dietary constituents despite the fact that they are not essential nutrients to the body.

- Adequate intake of dietary fiber prevents constipation, eliminates bacterial toxins, reduces GIT cancers, improves glucose tolerance and reduces plasma cholesterol.

- In general, vegetable oils are good sources for essential fatty acids while animal proteins are superior for the supply of essential amino acids.

- The biological value (BV) of protein represents the percentage of absorbed nitrogen retained in the body. The BV for egg protein is 94 while that of rice is 68.

- The recommended dietary allowance (RDA) of nutrients depends on the sex and age, besides pregnancy and lactation in the women.

- The habit of consuming mixed diet by man is largely responsible to enhance the nutritive value of foods, besides preventing several nutritional deficiencies (e.g., amino acids).

- Kwashiorkor and marasmus the two-extrme forms of protein-energy malnutrition in infants and pre-school children are highly prevalent in developing countries.

- Knowledge of the metabolism of xenobiotics is essential for the understanding of toxicology, pharmacology and drug addition.

- The body possesses the capability to get rid of the foreign substances by converting them into more easily excretable forms.

- Detoxification is not necessarily associated with the conversion of toxic into non-toxic compounds. For instance methanol is metabolized to more toxic formaldehyde.

- Detoxification primarily occurs in the liver through one or more of the reactions namely oxidation, reduction, hydrolysis and conjugation.

- British antilewisite (BAL) a compound developed during Second World War was used to detoxify certain poisons.

- Prostaglandins synthesized in almost all the tissues (exception erythrocytes) of the body act as local hormones.

- PGs perform diversified biochemical functions. These include lowering of blood pressure, inhibition of gastric HCl secretion, decrease in imunological response and induction of labor.

- Over production of PGs causes symptoms such as pain, fever, vomiting, nausea, inflammation etc. Aspirin/ibuprofen/corticosteroid administration inhibits PG synthesis and relieves these symptoms.

- Platelet aggregation that may lead to thrombosis is promoted by thromboxanes and prostaglandins E_1 and inhibited by prostacyclins.

- Leukotrienes are implicated in hypersensitivity (allergy) and asthma.

- Consumption of fish foods containing the unsaturated fatty acid namely eicosapentaenoic acid is advocated to prevent heart attacks.

- Biological membranes are relatively impermeable protective barriers that provide a connecting link between the cell (or its organelle) and its environment.

- The cells must contain high K^+ and low Na^+ concentrations for their survival. $Na^+ - K^+$ pump, which consumes a major protein of the cellular metabolic energy (ATP), is responsible for this.

- Ouabain inhibits $Na^+ - K^+$ ATPase ($Na^+ - K^+$ pump). It is extracted from the seeds of an African shrub and used as poison to tip the hunting arrows by the tribals.

- The transport of certain amino acids and sugars in to the cells occurs through a Na^+ co-transport system.

- Regulation of gene expression to adapt to the changes in the environment is a remarkable property of the living cells.

- The growth, development and differentiation of an organism involve complex mechanisms, which, ultimately depend on gene regulation.

- The housekeeping genes or constituents genes are expressed at almost a constant rate in the cells and they are not subjected to regulations, e.g., the enzymes of Krebs cycle.

- The capacity of the body to produce 10 billions (10^{10}) antigen specific immunoglobins is due to gene rearrangement.

- Knowledge on gene regulation helps in the understanding and control of several diseases, including cancer.

- Diabetes affects about 2 – 3% of the population and is a major cause of blindness, renal failure, heart attack and stroke.

- Diabetic ketoacidosis is frequently encountered in severe uncontrolled diabetics. The management includes administration of insulin, fluids and potassium.

- The hypoglycemic drugs commonly used in diabetic patients include tolbutamide, gibenclamide and acetohexamide.

- Measurement of glycated hemoglobin (HbA_1c) serves as a marker for diabetic control.

- The incidence of cancer increases as age advances more than 70% of the new cases occurring in persons over 60.

- Chemical carcinogens cause about 80% of the human cancers.

- The products of oncogenes (growth, GTP-binding proteins) have been implicated in the development of cancer. Antioncogenes apply breaks and regulate the cell proliferation.

- The physical and chemical agents, viruses and mutations result in the activation of oncogenes causing carcinogenesis.

- The abnormal products of tumor cells, referred to as tumor markers, (CEA, AFP, PSA) are useful, for the diagnosis and prognosis of cancer.

- AIDS is a global disease with an alarming increase in the incidence of occurrence. By 2020 AD, more than 10 crore people are likely to be affected by AIDS.

- Homosexuality (predominantly in men) and intravenous drug abuse are the major factors in the risk of AIDS transmission.

- The patients of AIDS are destined to die (within 5 – 10 years after infection), since there is no cure. However, administration of certain drugs (AZT, DDI) prolongs life.

- The clinical manifestations of AIDS are directly or indirectly related to immunosuppression (mostly due to reduced CD_4 cells). AIDs patients are freely exposed to all sorts of infections (viral, bacterial, fungal).

- Hemolysis of RBC, action of purgatives and edema due to hypoalbuminemia are related to osmosis. Polyuria observed in diabetics is due to osmotic diuresis.

- The acidic nature of gastric juice (high H) can be explained by Donnan membrane equilibrium.

- Dipalmitoyl lecithin is a lung surfactant that maintains low surface tension in the alveoli and facilitates the exchange of gases.

- Radioisotopes, besides being used in biochemical research are employed in the diagnosis and treatment of cancers.

- Separation of serum proteins and lipoproteins by electrophoresis is frequently employed to detect the associated abnormalities, e.g., multiple myeloma, lipoprotein disorders.

- Centrifuge, colorimeter and flame photometer are indispensable tools even in a small clinical laboratory. Centrifuge is useful for the separation of serum (or plasma) while colorimeter and flame photometer are essential for estimation of a wide variety of compounds in biological fluids.

- Radioimmunoassay and ELISA have tremendous applications in the diagnosis of hormonal disorders, cancers and therapeutic monitoring of dugs.

- Monoclonal antibodies produced by hybridoma technology are in use for the early detection of pregnancy diagnosis and treatment of cancers.

11

CAN YOU IDENTIFY WHO I AM?

Sr. No.	Statement /Specific function (S)	Who I am?
1.	Some eat to live and some live to eat but my function is to cater for all	Nutrition
2.	Complex is the ingested food, but digested to simpler products, absorbed by intestinal mucosal cells, assimilated and utilized by all cells	Natural food material
3.	I am the unit of biological activity, organized into subcellular organelles, assigned to each are specific duties, thus I truly represent life	Cell
4.	We are polyhydroxyaldehydes or ketones, classified into mono; oligo- and polysaccharides, held together by glycosidic bonds	Carbohydrates
5.	With water, I say Touch me not, to the tongue, I am tasteful, within limits, I am dutiful, in excess, I am dangerous	Lipids/Fats
6.	We transaminate and deaminate to liberate ammonia, that is detoxified in the liver to end product urea, greatly improvement to body are our nitrogen products, carbon skeleton is for glucose, fat or fuel.	Amino acids
7.	We are the basis of structure and function of life, composed of twenty amino acids, the building blocks, organized into primary, secondary, tertiary and quaternary structures, classified as simple, conjugated and derived proteins.	Proteins
8.	We are the catalysts of the living world, protein in nature and in action specific, rapid and accurate, huge in size but with small active centers, highly exploited for disease diagnosis in lab centers.	Enzymes
9.	We are for growth, health and welfare of organisms, discharge our duties directly or through coenzymes, deficiency symptoms are our alert signals, satisfied we shall be with additional supplements	Vitamins
10.	I am the chemical basis of life and heredity, organized into genes that control every function, composed of repeating units of deoxyribonucleotides, arranged in a double helix, held by hydrogen bonds	DNA
11.	I am the red of food, responsible for respiration, deliver O_2 to tissues and return CO_2 to lungs, influenced by factors pH, BPG and Cl^- in my functions, disturbed in my duties structural abnormalities	Hemoglobin
12.	I am the energy currency of the cell, continuous consumption and regeneration is my thrill, without me, all biochemical functions come to a standstill, existence of life is unimaginable without my will	ATP

Sr. No.	Statement /Specific function (S)	Who I am?
13.	Consumed through diet and produced in the body, participate in innumerable cellular functions; implicated in several health complications and blamed I am for no fault of mine.	Cholesterol
14.	We are the chemical messengers of the body, diversified in our structure and function, act either directly or through messengers, growth, health and welfare is our motto	Hormones
15.	Functional units of DNA, we are ultimate for all cellular activities, tailored to express as per tissue demands, mystery of our molecular action awaits unfolding	Genes
16.	Test tube technique of DNA amplification, I am capable of producing millions of copies in hours, with ease, accuracy, specificity and sensitivity, no wonder, I have revolutionized genetic engineering	PCR
17.	A technique I am separating mixture of compounds, to isolate, identify, characterized molecules as desired, working on the principles of adsorption, partition, ion-exchange, I am key biochemical tool in laboratory experimentation	Chromatography
18.	I am the most feared disease of the world, due to a retrovirus causing immunodeficiency, with no cure in sight, except prevention, I challenge the scientists worldwide to conquer me	AIDs

REFERENCES

Bonner, J. and Varner, J.E. (1969). *Plant Biochemistry*. Vol. I and Vol. II. Academic Press, New York.

Campbell, R.W. and Howell, J.A. (1995). *Comprehensive Biotechnology*. Pergamon Press, Oxford.

Conn, E.E. and Stumpf, P.K. (1976). *Outlines of Biochemistry*. John Wiley and Sons Inc. New York.

Dietrich Knorr, (1987). *Food Biotechnology*. Marcel Dekker, INC. New York.

Garrett, R.H. and Grisham, C.M. (1995). *Biochemistry*. Saunders College Publishing, New York.

Garrow, J.S. and James, W.P. (1998). *Human Nutrition and Dietetics*. Churchill Living Stone, Edinburgh.

Goodwin, T.W. and Mercer, E.I. (1972). *An Introduction to Plant Biochemistry*. Pergamon Press, Oxford.

Gupta, P.K. (2000). *Elements of Biochemistry*. Rastogi Publications, Meerut, India,

Gupta, M.L. and Jangir, M.L. (2002). Cell Biology: *Fundamentals and Applications*. Agribios, Jodhapur, India.

Khan, A.A. (1977). *Physiology and Biochemistry of Seed Dormancy and Germination*. North Holland Publishing Company, Oxford.

Lehninger, A.L. (1993). *Principles of Biochemistry*. CBS Publishers and Distributors, New Delhi.

Lehninger, A.L., Nelson, P. L. and Cox, M.M. (1993), (2nd edition). *Principles of Biochemistry*. CBS Publishers, New Delhi.

Lohar, P.S. (2007). *Biotechnology*. MJP Publisher 44, Nallathambi Street, Triplicane, Chennai-600 005

Prince, N.L. and Stevens, L. (1993). *Fundamentals of Enzymology*. Oxford Scientific, Oxford.

Plumer, D.T. (1971). *An Introductory to Practical Biochemistry*. Mc-Graw Hill Pub. Co., New York.

Rehm, H. J. and Reed, G. (1997). *Biotechnology*. Vol. I and Vol. II. Verlg Chemic Weinheim, USA.

Sadasivam, S. and Manikam, A. 1992. *Biochemical Methods for Agricultural Sciences*. Wiley Eastern Limited, New Delhi.

Satyanarayana, U. 2006. *Biochemistry*. Books and Allied (P) Ltd. Kolkata.

Singh, B.D. 2000. *Biotechnology*. Kalayani Publisher, Ludhiana.

Styer, L. (1994). 4th edition. *Biochemistry*. Freeman, W.H. and Company, New York.

Talwar, G.P. (1980). *Text Book of Biochemistry and Human Biology*. Prentice Hall of India, New Delhi.

Trueman, P. 2007. *Nutritional Biochemistry*. MJP Publisher 44, Nallathambi Street, Triplicane, Chennai-600 005

Thimmaiah, S.K. 1999. *Standard Methods of Biochemical Analysis*. Kalyani Publishers, New Delhi–110002

Veerakumari, L. 2007. *Biochemistry*. MJP Publisher 44, Nallathambi Street, Triplicane, Chennai-600 005

West, E.S. Todd, W.R., Mason, H.S. and Bruggan, T.V. 1968. *Textbook of Biochemistry*. Macmillan Company, New York.

White, A., Handler, P. and Smith, E.L. (1978). *Principles of Biochemistry*. Mc-Graw-Hill Kogakusha Ltd., Tokyo.

Wilson, K. and Goulding, K.H. (1992). 3rd edition. *A Biologist's Guide to Principles and Techniques of Practical Biochemistry*. Cambridge University Press, Cambridge.

PART–B

BIOTECHNOLOGY

1

DISCOVERIES

A. Chronological Development in Biotechnology

S. No.	Activity	Year
1.	Yeasts used to make wine and beer	Before 6000 BC
2.	Yeasts used for making leavened bread	About 4000 BC
3.	Sewage treatment systems using microbes developed/established	About 1910 AD
4.	Large scale production of acetone, butanol and glycerol using bacteria	1912–14
5.	Large scale production of penicillin	1944
6.	Mining of uranium with the aid of microbes (Canada)	1962
7.	First successful genetic engineering experiments	1973
8.	Marketing of human food of fungal origin (UK)	1980
9.	The use of monoclonal antibodies for diagnosis approved in U.S.A.	1981
10.	Approved for the use of insulin produced by genetically engineered microbes (GEMs) USA and UK	1983
11.	Animal interferons, produced by GEMs, approved for the protection of cattle against diseases.	1984
12.	Release of the first GM crop, herbicide resistant tobacco	1986
13.	First successful field trial of GM cotton herbicide resistant	1990
14.	FlavourSavr tomato becomes the first GM food approved for sale	1994
15.	Development in sequencing of *Arabidopsis thaliana* genome	2001
16.	Draft was prepared for sequencing of rice genome	2002

B. Discoveries

Year	Name of the Scientist	Discovery
1902	Haberlandt	First attempt of plant tissue culture; Father of plant tissue culture
1904	Hanning	Embryo culture of selected crucifers
1922	Knudson	A symbiotic germination of orchid seeds *in vitro*
1926	Went, F.W.	Identified growth promoting substance in Avena coleoptiles
1934	White	Successful establishment of root culture
1939	Gautheret, Nobecourt and White	Successful establishment of continuously growing callus cultures

Contd...

Year	Name of the Scientist	Discovery
1941	Van Overbeek	Coconut milk used for the first time in Datura tissue culture and a cell division factor detected in it.
1941	Braun	In Vitro culture of crown gall tissues
1942	Gautheret	Observation of secondary metabolites in plant callus cultures
1944	Skoog	*In vitro* adventitious shoot formation in tobacco
1951	Nitsch	Culture of excised ovaries *in vitro*
1952	Morel and Martin	Meristem culture to obtain virus-free plants in Dahlias
1953	Tulecke	Production of haploid callus of the gymnosperm *Ginkgo biloba* from pollen
1955	Miller et al.	Discovered kinetin a cell division hormone
1957	Skoog and Miller	Concept of regulation of organogenesis by changing the ratio of auxin:cytokinin
1959	Reinert and Steward	Regeneration of somatic embryos from callus clumps and cell suspensions of *Daucus carota*
1960	Cocking	Enzymatic digestion of cell walls to obtain large number of protoplasts
1960	Kanta	First test tube fertilization in *Papaver rhoeas*
1960	Morel	Orchid propagation by meristem culture
1962	Murashige and Skoog	Development of Murashige and Skoog nutrition medium
1964	Guha and Maheshwari	Production of first haploid plants from microspore culture of *Datura*
1965	Vasil and Hildebrandt	Differentiation of tobacco plants from a single isolated cell
1966	Meselson and Yuan	Restriction endonuclease term coined for a class of enzymes involved in cleaving DNA
1970	Power et al.	First protoplast fusion
1970	Smith	Discovery of first restriction endonuclease in *Haemophillus influenzae* Rd. It was later purified and named Hindi
1971	Takebe et al.	First regeneration of plants from protoplasts
1972	Carlson et al.	First report of regeneration of somatic hybrid plant through protoplast fusion in two species of *Nicotiana*
1972	Berg et al.	First recombinant DNA molecule produced using restriction enzymes
1972	Lobban and Kaiser	Use of DNA ligase to join the two fragments thus giving rise to recombinant DNA
1972	Temin	Discovery of reverse transcriptase, a wonderful enzyme which allows genetic information to flow in the reverse form

Contd...

Year	Name of the Scientist	Discovery
1973	Pierik et al.	Cytokinin found capable of Gerbera
1974	Reinhard	Bio-transformation in plant tissue cultures
1974	Zaenen et al. and Larebeke et al.	Discovery that the tumour inducing principle of Agrobacterium lies in the Ti plasmid
1976	Seibert	Shoot initiation from cryopreserved shoot apices of carnation
1976	Bomhoff et al.	Octopine and nopaline synthesis and breakdown found to be genetically controlled by the Ti plasmid of *A. tumefaciens.*
1977	Chilton et al.	Successful integration of the Ti plasmid DNA from *A. tumefaciens* in plants
1978	Melchers et al.	Somatic hybridization between distantly related species like tomato and potato, resulting in pomato
1978	Tabata et al.	Commercial production of shikonin through plant cell culture
1979	Marton et al.	Co-cultivation procedure developed for transformation of plant protoplasts with Agrobactrium
1980	Alfermann et al.	Use of immobilized whole cells for bio-transformation of digitoxin into digoxin
1980	Zambryski et al.	Studies on the structure of T-DNA cloning the complete EcoRI digest to Ti tobacco crown gall DNA into a phase vector, thus allowing the isolation of T-DNA border sequence
1981	Larkin and Scowcroft	Introduction of the term somaclonal variation
1982	Zimmermann	Electrofusion of protoplasts
1983	Herrera-Estrella L, Depicker A, Van Montagu M and Schell J.	First GM plant is created; a tobacco plant resistant to an antibiotic
1983	Kary Mullis	The idea of a polymerize chain reaction (PCR), a chemical DNA amplification process conceived
1984	De Block et al. and Horsch et al.	Transformation of tobacco with Agrobacterium; transgenic plants developed
1987	Sanford et al. and Klein et al.	Development of biolistic gene transfer method for plant transformation
1987	Barton et al.	Isolation of Bt gene from bacterium (*Bacillus thuringiensis*)
1997	Blattner et al.	Sequencing of *E. coli* genome
2001	Potrykus	Development of genetically engineered "Golden Rice".

2

ABBREVIATIONS

Short Form	Full Form
2, 4-D	2, 4-Dichlorophenoxyacetic acid
2-ip	Isopentenyl adenine
5-BUdR	5-Bromodeoxyuridine
Ab	Antibody
ABA	Abscisic acid
ACC	1-Aminocyclopropane-1-carboxylic acid
ACC	Aminocyclopropane carboxylic acid
ACMV	African cassava mosaic virus
ADA	Adenosine deaminase
ADP	Adenosine diphosphate
Ag	Antigen
AG-LCR	Asymmetric gap ligase chain reaction
AGP	Araribinogalactan protein
ANF	Atrial natriuretic factor
ARS	Autonomously replicating sequences
ARS	Autonomous replicating sequence
ATCC	American Type Culture Collection
ATL	Adult T-cell Leukemia
ATP	Adenosine triphosphate
AZT	Azidothymidine
BAC	Bacterial artificial chromosome
BCG	Bacillus of Calmette Guerien
BHC	Benzene hexachloride
BMV	Brome mosaic virus

Short Form	Full Form
BOD	Biochemical oxygen demand
bp	Base pairs
BPV	Bovine papilloma virus
CaMV	Cauliflower mosaic virus
CaOCL	Calcium hypochloride
CBD	Convention on Biological diversity
CCMV	Chrysanthmum chlorotic mottle virus
cDNA	Complementary DNA
cDNA	Copy DNA or Complementary DNA
CDR	Complement determining region
CEA	Carcinoembryonic antigen
CEN	Centromere
CFSTR	Continuous flow stirred tank reactor
CGT	Cyclodextrin glucosyltransferase
CH	Constant region of heavy chain (antibodies)
CHEFE	Countour clamped homogeneous electric field electrophoresis
CHS	Chalcone synthase
CL	Constant region of light chain (antibodies)
cM	CentiMorgan
CMS	Cytoplasmic male sterility
CMV	Cucumber mosaic virus
COD	Chemical oxygen demand
cos	Cohesive sequence
COS	Cv1 origin of SV40 (Cv1 is a monkey cell line)
CP	Coat protein
cpDNA	Chlooroplast DNA
CpG	Cyclopentadienyl guanosine
CPMB	Center for plant Molecular Biology
C-region	Constant region
CSIR	Council for Scientific and Industrial Research

Short Form	Full Form
CSL	Corn Steep Liquor
CSV	Chrysanthemum stunt virus
dATP	Deoxyadenosine triphosphate
DBT	Department of Biotechnology
dCTP	Deoxycytidine triphosphate
ddATP	2′, 3′-dideoxyadenosine triphosphate
ddCTP	2′, 3′-deoxycytidine triphosphate
ddGTP	2′, 3′-dideoxyguanosine triphosphate
DDT	Dichlorodimethyltetracetic acid
ddTTP	2′, 3′-dideoxythymidine triphosphate
DFR	Dihydroflavanol 4-reductase
dGTP	Deoxyguanosine triphosphate
DH	Doubled haploid
DHFR	Dihydrofolate reductase
DHK	Dihydrokaempferol
DHZ	Dihydrozeatin
DIMBOA	2,4-Dihydroxy-7-methoxy-1, 4-benzoxazin-3-one
DME	Dulbecco's enriched modification of minimal essential medium
DMSO	Dimethyl sulphoxide
DNase	Doxyribonuclease
DOPE	Dioleoyl phosphatidylethanolamine
DPD	Diffusion pressure deficit
DSP	Downstream processing
DTA	Diphtheria Toxin A Chain
EBR	Fluidized bed reactor
EDTA	Ethylene diamine tetra-acetic acid
EFE	Ethylene forming enzyme
EGF	Epidermal Growth Factor
EIA	Enzyme immuno assay
ELISA	Enzyme liked immunosorbent assay

Short Form	Full Form
EMIT	Enzyme multiple immuno assay technique
EPO	Erythropoietin
EPR	Electron paramagnetic resonance
EPSP	Enol pyruval shikimate phosphate
EPSPS	5-enolpyruvyl-3-phosphoshikimic acid synthase
ER	Endoplasmic reticulum
ES	Embryonic stem cells
ESPS	5-enolpyruvyl shikimate-3-phosphate synthase
EST	Expression sequence tags
ETS	Electron transport system
FAB	Fragment with antigen binding (of antibodies)
FACS	Fluorescence activated cell sorter
FAD	Fluorescein diacetate
Fc	Crystal forming fragment (of antibodies)
FDA	Fluoresce in diacetate
FGF	Fibroblast growth factor
FID	Fluorescence immuno assay
FISH	Fluorescence *in situ* hybridization
FLV	Feline leukemia virus
FMD	Foot and mouth disease
FR	Framework region
FSH	Follicle stimulating hormone
GA_3	Gibberellic acid
GEM	Genetically engineered micro-organism
GFP	Green fluorescent protein
G-LCR	Gap-ligase chain reaction
GM	Genetically modified
GOGAT	Glutamate synthase
GOX	Glyphasate oxidoreductase
GR	Growth regulator

Short Form	Full Form
GTP	Guanosine triphosphate
HACCP	Hazard analysis critical control point
HACs	Human artificial chromosome
HART	Hybrid arrested translation
HAT medium	Hypoxanthine aminopterin and thymidine medium
HBsAg	Hepatitis B surface antigen
hCG	Human chorionic gonadotropin
HEPA	High efficiency particulate air filters
HEPA filter	High efficiency particulate air filter
HGF	Hepatocyte growth factor
HGH	Human growth hormone
HGPRT	Hypoxanthine-guanine phosphoribosyl transferase
HIV	Human immune deficiency syndrome
hMG	Human menopausal gonadotropin
hr	Hours
HSV	Herpes simplex virus
HSV-tk	Herpes simplex virus thymidine kinase
HTLV-1	Human T-cell leukemia lymphoma virus-1
IAA	Indole-3-acetic acid
IAM	Indole-3-acetamide
IARI	Indian Agricultural Research Institute
IBA	Indole-3-butyric acid
ICAR	Indian Council of Agricultural Research
ICGEB	International Centre for Genetic Engineering and Biotechnology
IEDCs	Induced embryogenic determined cells
Ig	Immunoglobulin
IGF	Insulin like growth factor
IL	Interleukin
IL-2	Interleukin-2
IMDM	Iscoves modified Dulbecco's medium

Short Form	Full Form
INF	Interferon
IP	Imbibitional pressure
IS	Insertion sequence
ISH	In situ hybridization
IV	Intermediate vector
IVRI	Indian Veterinary Research Institute
kb	Kilo base pairs
kg	Kilogram
l	Litre
LAK Cells	Lymphokine activated killer cells
LCR	Ligase chain reaction
LGL	Large granular lymphocyte
LH	Luteinising hormone
LN	Liquid nitrogen
LRE	Light response element
M	Molar (= gram molecular weight)
m mol 1^{-1}	Milli mole per liter
Mab	Monoclonal antibody
Mb	Mega base pairs (10^6 bp)
MEM	Eagles' minimal essential medium
min	Minutes
MLV	Moloney murine leukemia virus
mM	Milli molar (= mg molecular weight)
mol	Gram molecular weight
MS	Murashige and skoog medium
MSV	Maize streak virus
MTA	S-methyl thioadenosine
mtDNA	Mitochondrial DNA
MTOC	Microtubule organizing centers
Mtx	Methotrexate

Short Form	Full Form
NAA	Naphthalene acetic acid
NAD	Nicotinamide adenine dinucleotide
NADH	Nicotinamide adenine dinucleotide (reduced)
NaOCL	Sodium hypochloride
NBPGR	National Bureau of plant Genetic Resources
NBTB	National Biotechnology Board
NCL	National Chemical Laboratory
NDRI	National Dairy Research Institute
NGF	Nerve growth factor
NHI	Non-heme iron
NIL	Near isogenic lines
NIR	Near infrared spectroscopy
NK cells	Natural killer cells
NMR	Nuclear magnetic resonance
NPTII	Neomycin phosphotransferase
OSRV	Odontoglossum-ringspot virus
p.s.i.	Pounds per square inch
PALA	N-Phosphonacetyl-L-aspartate
PBR	Packed bed reactor
PC	Phosphatidyl choline
PCA	Packed cell volume
PCB's	Polychlorinated biphenyls
PCR	Polymerase chain reaction
PCR	Polymerase chain reactions
PDA	Potato dextrose agar
PDB	Paradichloro benzene
PDGF	Platelet-derived growth factor
PEDLs	Pre-embryogenically determined cells
PEG	Polyethylene glycol
PFGE	Pulsed field gel electrophoresis

Short Form	Full Form
Pg	Picogram
PG	Polygalacturonase
PGR	Plant Growth Regulators
PHB	Polyhydroxy butyrate
PHB	Polyhydroxy butyrate
PLA	Polylactic acid
PMSG	Pregnant mare serum gonadotropin
ppb	Parts per billion
ppm	Parts per million
PS	Pedigree selection
PVC	Polyvinyl carbonate
PVP	Polyvinyl pyrrolidon
PVS	Potato virus S
PVX	Potato virus X
PYAC	Yeast artificial yeast chromosome vector
QTL	Quantitative trait loci
QTL	Quantitative trait loci
r.p.m.	Revolutions per minute
RAPD	Random Amplified Polymorphic DNA
RAPD	Randomly amplified polymorphic DNAs
RFLP	Restriction fragment length polymorphism
RH	Relative humidity
RIA	Radio-immune assay
RNase	Ribonuclease
RNP	Ribonucleic protein
RSV	Rous sarcoma virus
RTF	Resistance transfer factor
RuBISCO	Ribulose 1,5-bisphosphate carboxylase/oxygenase
s	Seconds
SAM	S-adenosyl methionine

Short Form	Full Form
SAR	Systemic acquired resistant
SCID	Severe combined immune deficiency
SCP	Single cell protein
SE	Somatic embryo
SP	Suction pressure
SSBP	Single strand binding protein
SSD	Single cell protein
SSR	Short sequence repeats
STMS	Sequence tagged micro satellite sites
STR	Stirred tank reactors
STS	Sequence tagged sites
SV 40	Simian virus 40
TAV	Tomato aspermy virus
TBGRI	Tropical Botanical Garden and Research Institute
TCPP	Tissue culture pilot plant
T-DNA	Transferred DNA
TDZ	Thidiazuron
TERI	Tata Energy Research Institute
TGF-β	Transforming growth factor β
Tk	Thymidine kinase
TMGMV	Tobacco mild green mosaic virus
TMV	Tobacco mosaic virus
TNF	Tumour necrosis factor
TobRV	Tobacco ringspot virus
ToMV	Tobacco mosaic virus
TP	Turgor pressure
tPA	Tissue plasminogen activator
TTC	2,3,5-Triphenyl tetrazolium chloride
UNO	United Nations Organization
UV	Ultraviolet (light)

Short Form	Full Form
V/V	Volume by volume
VH	Variable region of heavy chain (antibodies)
VL	Variable region of light chain (antibodies)
VNTR	Variable number tandem repeats
VP 1,2 or 3	Virion protein 1, 2 or 3
V-region	Variable region (in antibodies)
VS	Volatile solids
VV	Vaccinia virus
W/V	Weight by volume
W/W	Weight by weight
WDA	Wheat dwarf virus
WP	Wall pressure
WPM	Woody plant medium
x	Genomic chromosome number
XGPRT	Xanthine-guanine phosphoribosyl transferase
YAC	Yeast artificial chromosome
YCP	Yeast centromere plasmids
YEP	Yeast episomal plasmids
YIP	Yeast integrative plasmids
YRP	Yeast replicating plasmids

3

TERMINOLOGY

Term	Definition
Agrobacteriam rhizogenes	A species of gram-negative rod shaped soil bacteria closely related to *Agrobacterium tumefaciens*; often contains copies of a large plasmid, designated Ri. Ri plasmids are similar to the Ti plasmids of A. tumefaciens. A Ri-containing strain can cause a tumorous growth known as hairy root disease in certain plants.
Agrobacterium tumefaciens	A species of gram-negative, rod shaped soil bacteria contains copies of a large plasmid, designated Ti. A Ti-containing strain can infect the stems of many plants and form crown gall tumors.
Aliquot	An exact fractional sample or portion of a whole (used especially of solutions).
Anneal	To hybridize nucleic acid molecules by means of complementary base pairing between two strands of DNA or between DNA and RNA.
Antibiotic	A substance produced by one organism, that inhibits or kills another organism, usually bacteria. Antibiotics typically are active against bacteria and are produced by fungi or streptomycetes.
Antisense gene	An engineered gene placed in inverted orientation relative to a promoter which when transcribed, produces a transcript complementary to the mRNA from the normal orientation of the gene.
Antiserum	Blood serum containing specific antibodies against an antigen.
Aseptic	Characterized by absence of contaminating fungi, bacteria, viruses, mycoplasms, and other micro-organisms (e.g., in cultures).

Term	Definition
Autoradiography	A method for determining the presence and location of radioactivity labeled molecules by their effect in creating an image on a photographic emulsion, usually X-ray film, by activating the silver when the film is developed. Autoradiography is commonly used to determine whether a radioactive probe molecule has hybridized to denatured DNA or RNA following Southern or Northern transfers, respectively or in colony hybridization procedures.
Base	One of the four chemical units on the DNA or RNA molecule, which according to their order and pairing, represent the different amino acids. In DNA the four bases are adenine (A), cytosine (C), guanine (G) and thymine (T). The purine bases are adenine and guanine; the pyrimidine bases are cytosine, thymine and uracil.
Base pair	Two nucleotide bases on different strands of the nucleic acid molecule that from hydrogen bonds between them. The bases can pair in a single way only; adenine with thymine (in DNA) or uracil (in RNA) and guanine with cytosine.
Biotechnology	Development of products by a biological process requiring engineering technologies, such as fermentation or controlled environments or utilizing current technologies (such as recombinant DNA techniques) for the modification and improvement of biological systems including plants.
	Fusion of biology and technology.
	It consists of the controlled use of biological agents such as microorganisms or cellular components for beneficial use.
	It is the integrated use of biochemistry, microbiology and engineering sciences in order to achieve technological application of the capabilities of microorganisms cultured tissues/cells and parts thereof.
	It is controlled and deliberate application of simple biological agents.
	It consists the application of biological organisms, systems or processes.

Term	Definition
	It consists of biochemistry, microbiology, chemistry, genetics, molecular biology, immunology, cell and tissue culture & physiology as well as engineering.
Biotechnology Old	The processes, which are based on the natural capabilities of microorganisms, are commonly considered as old biotechnology.
Biotechnology New	Non-natural capabilities of microorganisms for well-being of human.
Blot	To transfer DNA, RNA or proteins, usually from an electrophoretic gel to an immobilizing matrix such as nitrocellulose, or nylon membranes. Also the autoradiograph obtained from hybridization analysis after the transfer is called blot.
Blunt ends	The double strand DNA ends left on a restriction fragment by most Type I and some Type II restriction endonucleases. These paired regions are not readily available for hybridization with other fragments during gene cloning experiments.
bp	The symbol for base pair, a measure of the size of a double strands nucleic acid (1000 bp = 1 kbp).
CAT box or CATT box	A conserved sequence found as part of the promoter region 75 bp upstream of the transcription start point of the protein encoding genes of many eukaryotic organisms.
cDNA	Complementary DNA; single strand DNA complementary to an RNA molecule. cDNA is synthesized in vitro from the RNA primer by the enzyme reverse transcriptase. For cloning purpose, double-stranded DNA can be made from the cDNA template by the enzyme DNA polymerase and inserted into an appropriate vector.
cDNA cloning	The use of cDNA to clone the coding sequence of a gene or sets to genes by starting with mRNA. The cDNA from mature processed transcripts does not contain introns, the presence of which could act to prevent expression of plant or animal cDNAs when attached to a suitable promoter and cloned into a host organism such as bacteria or yeast.

Term	Definition
Chimeric gene	A recombinant gene that contains sequences from more than one source, such as a coding sequence from one source and a promoter region from another.
Chromosome	The structural component in the cell that carries the gene; composed of DNA and proteins.
Clone	A population of recombinant DNA molecules all carrying the same inserted sequence or a population of cells derived from a single cell by mitoses or a population of plants derived from a single cell by vegetative propagation (e.g., by cuttings, bulbs, tubers, rhizomes, stolons or meristem culture) or to use recombinant DNA techniques to insert a particular gene or other DNA sequence into a vector molecule.
Coding sequence	That portion of a gene, which derived, specifies the amino acid sequence of its protein product. Non-coding sequences of genes include control regions, such as promoters, operators, enhancers, terminators and introns.
Constitutive	An organism is said to be constitutive for the production of an enzyme or other protein if the cells under all physiological conditions always produce that protein; i.e. the gene is always on.
Construction of genomic library	From the total genomic DNA of an organism (by extracting). The minimum number of colonies in a genomic library constructed with 20 Kb (kilo base pairs) inserts for a 99% probability of all the genomic sequences being represented would be 1157 for *E. coli* (genome of 3.75×10^3 Kb), 3462 for yeast (genome, 1.5×10^4 Kb), 38000 for Drosophila (genome, 1.65×10^5 Kb), and 690819 for man (genome, 3×10^6 Kb).
Copy number	The number of plasmid molecules per cell or the number of times a specific gene is present per haploid genome.

Term	Definition
Cotransformation	A technique in which host cells are incubated with two plasmids, one containing a selectable marker gene and the other containing a gene that cannot be identified by direct selection. Cells selected for the presence of the marker gene are competent for DNA uptake and are more likely to have also been transformed with the second plasmid, thereby reducing the number of cells that must be screened by other means (such as probe hybridization for the second gene).
Crown gall	A tumor formed predominantly on the stems of broadleaved plant when infected with *Agrobacterium tumefaciens* containing a Ti-plasmid. Part of the Ti-plasmid (T-DNA) is transferred into the genome of the affected plant cells due to action of the Ti-plasmid *vir* genes. Expression of T-DNA genes for auxin and cytokinin synthesis cause gall formation even in the absence of the bacterium. Whole plants can sometimes be regenerated from crown gall tissue and some of these still contain T-DNA.
Denaturation	The breakdown of the secondary, tertiary structure of a protein or nucleic acid by physical or chemical means. More specifically, the conversion of a double-strand nucleic acid to the single stranded state by destruction the double-stranded state.
DNA polymerase	One of several enzymes, which synthesize a new DNA strand complementary to a template strand by adding nucleotides one at a time to a 3' –OH end.
Electroblotting	The electrophoretic transfer of macromolecules (DNA, RNA or protein) from a gel in which they have been separated onto a support matrix such as a nitrocellulose sheet. The procedure is an alternative to the capillary transfer used in techniques such as Southern and Northern blotting.
Electrophoresis	A technique for separating different types of molecules based on their patterns of movement in an electrical field.
Electroporation	Application of an electrical current across a membrane (as in a protoplast), including temporary pores & permitting uptake of molecules, organelles etc., or fusion of neighboring membranes.

Term	Definition
End labeling	The linking of a radioactive atom such as ^{32}P to the end of a DNA or RNA molecule by a ligation reaction carried out by an enzyme such as T4 polynucleotide kinase.
Endonuclease	An enzyme that cleaves within the polynucleotide chain.
Exon	That part of the gene, which is transcribed and represented in the mature mRNA after transcript processing and removal of sequences corresponding to introns. The protein product thus represents the exon sequence information.
Expression vector	A cloning vector containing an effective promoter such that a gene inserted at a specific site will be efficiently transcribed and translated into a protein product.
Extrachromosomal	Located elsewhere than the nuclear chromosome, such as in an organelle or on a plasmid.
Gel	The inert matrix used for the electrophoretic separation of nucleic acids or proteins.
Gene	The physical and functional unit of heredity that encodes a functional protein or RNA molecule. More specifically, a segment of chromosome, plasmid, or DNA molecule that includes regions preceding and following the coding region and possibly introns located between exons.
Genetic engineering	The use of *in vitro* techniques to produce DNA, molecules containing novel combinations of genes or other sequences in living cells that make them capable of producing new substances or performing new functions.
Genomic library	It is a collection of plasmid clones or phage lysates containing recombinant DNA molecules.
β-glucuronidase	Reporter gene from *E. coli*; a hydrolase that catalyzes the cleavage of a wide variety of β-glucuronides. One of the most commonly used is 5-bromo-4-chloro-3-indolyl glucuronide (X-GLUC), which shows dark blue colour in transformed cells and tissues.

Term	Definition
Homology	The extent to which two nucleic acid molecules have the same nucleotide sequence or two proteins have the same amino acid sequence. Homology can be determined by direct comparisons of sequence data, or estimated by DNA-DNA or DNA-RNA hybridization. The degrees of identity between chromosomes or chromosome segments also determine homology.
Hybridization	The paring of complementary DNA or RNA strands to give stable DNA-DNA or DNA-RNA duplexes. The efficiency of hybridization is a test of sequence homology.
Inducer	A small chemical molecule or a physical agent that increases transcription of specific genes when applied to cells, tissues, organs or organisms.
Inducible	The capability of a gene or its promoter to increase transcription when exposed to an inducing agent.
Insert	The piece of foreign DNA introduced into a vector molecule.
Insertion site	A unique restriction site in a vector DNA molecule into which foreign DNA can be inserted. The term also describes the position of integration of a transposable element.
Intensifying screen	A plastic sheet impregnated with a rare-earth compound such as calcium tungstate. The rare-earth compound absorbs beta radiation and emits light. When placed on one side of a piece of X-ray film with a radioactive sample on the other side, the intensifying screen will capture some of the beta emissions that pass through the film. The light emitted by the screen upon beta capture will blacken the X-ray film and enhance the sensitivity of the detection. It is used in Southern and Northern blotting experiments.
Intron	A DNA sequence within a gene that is transcribed, but is removed from the transcript by splicing together exon sequences on either side of it.
In Vitro	Carried out in sterile cultures. Outside the intact organism. Applied to various biological processes such as tissue culture and measurements, enzyme reactions; literally in glass.

Term	Definition
In Vivo	Occurring in a living whole organism, *i.e.*, in animal or plant.
Ligase	An enzyme, which forms a phosphodiester bond to link two adjacent bases separated by a nick in one strand of a double-stranded DNA. Ligases are also used to join two separated blunt to join two separated blunt end DNAs, and for the joining of RNA.
Miniprep	A small-scale preparation of plasmid or phage DNA commonly used after cloning to analyze the DNA sequence inserted into a cloning vector.
Nick	A break in DNA. More specifically the absence of a phosphodiester bond between adjacent nucleotides in one of the two strands of a DNA duplex.
Nick translation	A technique for radioactivity labeling a DNA molecule to high specific activity to produce a probe for use in nucleic acid hybridization. Random nicks or gaps are introduced into the probe DNA molecule using a limited DNase digest. The 5' to 3' exonuclease activity of DNA polymerase 1 enlarges the gaps and at the same time its polymerase activity fills in the gaps with α-labeled ^{32}P deoxynucleotide triphosphates to yield newly synthesized DNA stretches that are highly radioactive.
Nitrocellulose	A nitrated derivative of cellulose that is made into membrane filters of defined porosity such as 0.45 mm, 0.22 mm. These filters have a variety of uses in molecular biology, particularly in nucleic acid hybridization experiments, in which the nucleic acids are transferred from an agarose gel to a nitrocellulose filter.
Northern blot	The transfer of RNA from an electrophoretic gel to a filter so that it can be hybridized with a nucleic acid probe.
Nucleotide	A nucleic acid base bound to a sugar and a phosphate group, i.e., nucleoside with a phosphate group added.
Oligonucleotide	A short-chain nucleic acid molecule consisting of a small number of nucleotides.

Term	Definition
Organelle genome	The DNA of chloroplasts or mitochondria. The chloroplasts genome ranges in size from 120 to 200 kb, and the mitochondrial genome in higher plants ranges from 200 to > 2200 kb. These genomes exist as circular chromosomes lacking structural proteins and may be present in many copies per cell. Small linear or circular plasmids may also be present in mitochondria.
Plasmid	An autonomous, self-replicating extra chromosomal DNA, which is often circular. The size varies from < 1kb to > 300 kb and copy number per cell ranges from 1 to > 100; have genes for specific functions, such as antibiotic resistance.
Polyacrylamide gel electrophoresis	A method for separating nucleic acid or protein molecules. The molecules migrate through an inert gel matrix under the influence of an electric field; their mobility is a function of their net charge, size and shape. Sodium dodecyl sulfate polyacrylamide gel electrophoresis for separation of proteins according to size, a detergent such as sodium dodecyl sulfate is added to ensure that all molecules have a uniform charge.
Polymerase chain reaction (PCR)	An in vitro procedure to amplify the number of copies of a specific DNA sequence often found in rare abundance in a complex DNA source. Two single stranded synthetic oligonucleotides of defined sequence are required to prime synthesis of the source DNA sequence located between its sites of homology to the primers. Primers are annealed to denatured DNA and DNA polymerase from *Thermus aquaticus* is added to initiate synthesis of two complementary DNA strands by extension from the primers. The reaction mixture is alternately heated (to produce single stranded templates for the next round of synthesis) and then cooled (to allow synthesis to proceed). After the first few cycles, most new strands end at the primer from the previous synthesis. A sequence of a specific length and base sequence can be amplified many orders of magnitude and used for cloning, sequence analysis, and other molecular biology procedures.

Term	Definition
Primer	A short oligonucleotide that is paired with one strand of DNA and provides a free 3' hydroxy group required for initiation of DNA synthesis by DNA polymerase.
Probe	A defined nucleic acid sequence that has been labeled with a radioactive isotope or fluorescent dye. It is used to identify specific DNA or RNA molecules that have the complementary sequence. Also used to perform hybridization to detect a specific gene or transcript.
Promoter	A regulatory region of DNA near one of the two ends usually the 5" end of the coding sequence of agene or operon that binds RNA polymerase and directs the enzyme to the correct transcriptional start site.
Protoplast	A membrane-bound cell formed after the cell wall is removed from a microbial or plant cell by the action of pectinases and cellulases. Protoplasts are used to produce hybrid cells via fusion and to facilitate transformation through direct gene transfer.
Recombinant DNA	DNA molecules in which sequences that are not naturally continuous have been placed next to each other by *in vitro* manipulations. The different sequences placed within a recombinant DNA molecule frequently are obtained from entirely different organisms.
Regulatory gene	A gene, which acts to control the protein-synthesizing activity of other genes.
Restriction endonuclease	An endonuclease that recognizes a specific sequence of bases within double-stranded DNA. Type I restriction endonucleases bind to this recognition site but subsequently cut the DNA at approximately random sites, while Type III restriction endonucleases cut at about 25 bp from the recognition site. Type II restriction endonucleases both bind and cut within their recognition or target site. They may make the cuts in the two DNA strands exactly opposite one another and generate

Term	Definition
	blunt ends or they may make staggered cuts to generate sticky ends. Only Type II restriction endonucleases are used in recombinant DNA technology. Names for restriction endonucleases start with three italic letters identifying the source bacterium; subsequent letters (not italic) identify the strain or serotype; and capital roman numerals at the end of the name indicate enzyme Type I, II or III, Not all possible elements appear in every name. For example: EcoB is derived from strain B of *Escherichia coli*; Mbol is enzyme I from *Moraxella bevis*; BamHI is enzyme I from Strain H of *Bacillus amyloliquefaciens*; HindIII is enzyme III from Steriotyped of *Haemophillus infeunzae*.
Restriction fragment	An individual polynucleotide sequence produced by the digestion of DNA with a restriction endonulease.
Restriction site	The specific nucleotide sequence in DNA recognized by a Type II restriction endonucleases and within which it makes a double-stranded cut. Restriction sites usually comprise four or six base pairs and have bilateral symmetry. For example, 5'-G A G C T C-3' and 3'-C T C G A G-5'. The two strands may be cut directly opposite to one another to create blunt ends or in a staggered manner giving sticky ends, depending on the enzyme involved.
Ri Plasmid	A class of large, conjugative plasmids found in the soil bacterium *Agrobacterium rhizogenes*. A segment of the Ri plasmid (T-DNA) is found in the genome of tumor tissue from plants with hairy root disease.
RNA polymerase	An enzyme, which catalyzes the synthesis of RNA from a DNA template in the absence of a 3' primer molecule. A single RNA polymerase that synthesizes all classes of RNA molecules accomplishes transcription in prokaryotes. Eukaryotes have three RNA polymerases, with different transcriptional specificities: RNA polymerase I or A synthesizes the large rRNA; II or B synthesizes mRNA; III or C synthesizes tRNA and 5S rRNA species.

Term	Definition
Southern blot	A technique (designated after its inventor, E.M. Southern), which combines the resolving power of agarose gel electrophoresis with the sensitivity of nucleic acid hybridization. DNA fragments separated in an agarose gel are denatured *in situ* and then blotted by capillary action or electric field from the gel onto a nitrocellulose sheet or other binding matrix placed next to the gel. Single-stranded DNA binds to the nitrocellulose and is then available for hybridization with a ^{32}P-labeled or biotinylated, single-stranded DNA or RNA probe. The hybrids are detected by autoradiography; the case of ^{32}P or a colour change in the case of a biotinylated probe.
Splicing	Transcript processing by which intron sequences are removed from precursor RNA molecules and adjacent exon sequences are rejoined by ligation, in recombinant DNA terminology, splicing is also used to indicate the insertion of a DNA sequence into a vector molecule.
T-DNA	Transferred DNA; The segment of DNA from a Ti or Ri plasmid that is transferred from *Agarobacterium* to the genome of its plant host and causes tumor formation or root induction. Plants regenerated from Ti or Ri plasmid induced callus tissue can stably inherit the T-DNA. Foreign DNA inserted into the T-DNA can also be stably inherited.
TATA box	A highly conserved, AT-rich, 7-base sequence found about 25 bases prior to the transcription start site of RNA polymerase II transcribed eukaryotic genes. The TATA sequence facilitates, but is not essential for transcription.
Ti plasmid	A class of large, conjugative plasmids found in the soil bacterium *Agrobacterium tumefaciens* and responsible for the crown gall disease of broad-leaved plants. The T-DNA region on the Ti plasmid is inserted into the genome of infected host cells or plants, which makes Ti plasmids and T-DNA specifically useful for transformation of region genes into certain plants.

Term	Definition.
Transcript	The RNA product of gene. The primary transcripts initially synthesized by RNA polymerases must often be mature, functional mRNA, rRNA or tRNA species.
Transgenic	Of cells, cell cultures, plants or progeny: having received a foreign or modified gene by one of the various methods of transformation as described in this manual.
Transient expression	The short-term detectable expression of the product of a gene, which has been transferred into protoplasts, cells or plants. Marker genes on the DNA construct such as GUS or GFP–glucuronidase that are readily assayed in plant tissues are often used to determine whether DNA has been transferred into the cells. Transient expression indicates only that the marker gene is transcribed and translated in the cells assayed, and does not imply that the gene or DNA construct has been heritably incorporated into the plant genome.
Vector	The plasmid or phage chromosome used to carry cloned DNA in recombinant DNA experiments. A vector generally contains one or more unique restriction sites, is capable of autonomous replication in a defined host, and confers a well-defined, selectable phenotype on the host organism such as drug resistance.
Western blot	A procedure for transfer of proteins after separation on a polyacrylamide gel to a suitable immobilizing matrix such as a nitrocellulose sheet. The proteins attached to the support matrix can then be probed with a specific antibody to identify a particular protein species.

4

SHORT EXPLANATIONS

Difference between New and Old Biotechnology

Old Biotechnology	New Biotechnology
Man began employing microorganisms as early as 5000 BC for making wine, vinegar, curd, leavened bread etc. Some of these processes are so common and have become such an integral part of the usual kitchen technology of every home that we may even hesitate to refer anmal to them as biotechnology. Such an other processes, which are based on the natural capabilities of micro organisms etc., are commonly considered as old biotechnology.	Man has continued his quest for improving the natural capabilities of microorganisms with new capabilities. The development of recombinant DNA technology create highly valuable, novel and naturally non existent capabilities. Animal and plant cells and their components are being employed to generate valuable products. Crop varieties and breeds with entirely new and highly useful traits are being created with the help of recombinant DNA technology. These and many similar examples constitute the new biotechnology.

Scope and Importance of Biotechnology

In the following fields the biotechnology can make remarkable contributions:

1. Human health
2. Medicines
3. Animal health
4. Dairy Science
5. Animal husbandry
6. Chemicals and biochemicals
7. Fod Processing and beverages
8. Agriculture
9. Forestry
10. Horticulture and Floriculture
11. Environment
12. Renewable energy and fuels
13. Mining
14. Population control
15. Fisheries and aquaculture
16. Crimes and parentage disputes

Institutions established in India for working on Biotechnological Research Areas

An importance of biotechnology was highlighted in Indian Science Congress held at Mysore in 1982. Government of India constituted a National Biotechnology

Board (NBTB) to encourage and coordinate research activities in Biotechnology. The Department of Biotechnology was established within the Ministry of Science and Technology in 1986. Research centers for Biotechnology have been established at 1. Indian Agricultural Research Institute (IARI), New Delhi; 2. National Dairy Research Institute (NDRI) Karnal; and 3. Indian Veterinary Research Institute (IVRI), Izat Nagar. Department of Biotechnology, Indian Council of Agricultural Research (ICAR), New Delhi and Council for Scientific and Industrial Research (CSIR), New Delhi are also promoting research activities in biotechnology.

Advantages of Plant Biotechnology

1. Useful biochemical production (large scale cell cultures).

2. Rapid clonal multiplication (adventitious shoot/bulb/protocorm or SE regeneration, axillary bud proliferation).

3. Virus elimination (thermo-, cryo- or chem-therapy coupled with meristem culture).

4. Rapid development of homozygous lines by producing haploids (anther culture, ovary culture, interspecific hybridization).

5. Production/recovery of difficult to produce hybrids (embryo rescue in vitro pollination).

6. Germplasm conservation of vegetative reproducing plants or those producing recalcitrant seeds (cryo preservation slow growth cultures, DNA clones).

7. Genetic modification of plants (somaclonal variation, somatic hybridization, hybridization and gene transfer).

8. Creation of genome maps and use of molecular markers to assist conventional breeding efforts.

Biochemical production from cultured plants cells offers several advantages over their extraction from field grown plants; some of these are as follows.

1. It relieves pressure of over-exploitation/threat of extinction of natural populations of plant species, e.g., L. erythrorhizom.

2. In cases where plant material is limited in supply, e.g., Trichosanthes and/or the plants are slow growing, e.g., L. erythrorhizom, cultures offer a system of continuous supply.

3. In many cases cultured cells produce higher biochemical levels than the differentiated plant tissues, e.g., 20% (on dry weight basis) shikonin by Lithospermum cell cultures compared in 1.5% in roots.

4. Plants cells carry out many biotransformations.

5. Cells can be readily separated from the medium by simple filtration and stored at –30°C till the biochemicals are extracted.

Limitations

1. High production cost is the major disadvantage.

2. Many systems are difficult to improve upon mainly because of a lack of the basic knowledge of the biosynthetic routes. This knowledge is essential for enhancing the production levels to make the process economical.

3. Often cultured plant cells do not produce compounds of high value.

Somaclones resistant to specific disease:

Crop	Disease	Somaclones remark
Sugarcane	Fiji disease	More resistant to Fiji disease
Potato	Early blight Late blight	More resistant than parent clone. Resistant to race O
Apple	Scab	More resistant than parent variety

New crop varieties developed by anther culture or hybridization with *Hordeum bulbosum.*

Haploid production route	Crop	Varieties	Country
Anther culture	Rice	Tanfeng 1, Tan Fong 1, Hua Yu 1, Hua Yu 2, TaBe 78, Xin Xiu, Xhonghua 8, Xhonghua 9 etc.	China
Anther culture	Wheat	Hua Pei 1, Lung Hua 1, Jinghua 1, Yunhua 1, Yunhua 2, etc.	China
Anther culture	Wheat	Florin	Europe
Anther culture	Tobacco	Tan Yu 1, Tan Yu 2, Tan Yu 3 etc.	China
Anther culture	Tobacco	F 211	Japan
Hordeum bulbosum	Barley	Mingo, Gwylan	Canada

Role of Biochemistry in Plant Biotechnological Research

- Plant biotechnology is the use and manipulation of plants or the substances obtained from them, to make products of value to humanity.

  Integration of several disciplines: 1. Biochemistry 2. Genetics 3. Genetic engineering 4. Plant tissue culture 5. Microbiology 6. Molecular biology

- Progress in genetic engineering has been made possible due to the development of technology that allows scientists to isolate, identify and clone genes.

- Restriction endonucleases (also called restriction enzymes) are a group of enzymes that recognize specific nucleotide sequence in DNA, often 4 or 6 base pairs long and cut both strands of DNA within the recognition site.

- Joining or recombining DNA segments from different sources, which is catalyzed by enzyme DNA ligase, makes Recombinant DNA.

Plant Genetic Engineering and its Applications

- It involves transfer of genes from one organism to another. That gene must be correctly expressed at the right time and in the right organ, tissue or cell and must have the right function.

- In order to achieve the desired goal, it is essential to have the complete knowledge of the biochemical pathways, their regulation and enzymes involved.

- Genetic engineering means integrating one or more new genes so that a new enzyme will be made in transgenic plant.

- Genetically engineered plants are expected to influence all aspects of farming, food production and food processing industries.

- Based on the existing knowledge and utilizing available technologies, it is now possible to modulate plant functions either by the suppressing/ over expression of endogenous proteins or by introduction of genes encoding foreign proteins.

- Biochemistry plays an important role in biotechnology by explaining with following points.

1. **Herbicide tolerance**

   - Herbicides inhibit plant growth by blocking the biosynthesis of amino acids. These include glyphosate (N-phosphonomethyl-glycine), which inhibits the synthesis of aromatic amino acids (tryptophan, phenylalanine, tyrosine), the sulphonyl ureas and imidazolinones, which block branched chain amino acid biosynthesis; and phosphinothricin, which inhibits glutamine biosynthesis.

     Glyphosate tolerant transgenic plants of a large number of crops (beet, corn, cotton, lettuce, poplar, potato, rapeseed, soybean, tobacco, tomato, wheat) have already been field-tested and are entering agriculture.

   - 5-enolpyruvyl-3-phosphoshikimic acid synthase (EPSPS) and glyphasate oxidoreductase (GOX) Tolerant to glyphosate herbicide, this can be over come by transgenic plants.

2. **Insect-pest resistance**

    *   Transgenic tomato, tobacco, potato, maize and cotton plants resistant to lepidopteran insect pests have been developed by transforming them with the genes from *Bacillus thuringiensis* (B.t.) encoding insecticidal proteins.

    *   Other proteins called lectins bind to proteins in the gut and interfere with the absorption of nutrients in the small intestine.

    *   Defense proteins are the inhibitors of digestive enzymes protease inhibitors and amylase inhibitors.

    *   A trypsin inhibitor gene from cowpea which imparts resistance to a beetle herbivore by interfering with its digestion when introduced into tobacco imparted resistance to bud worm.

3. **Disease resistance**

    *   Plants can be immunized against viruses in the same way that the people are immunized against bacterial disease (cross-protection in plants).

    *   The approach followed is introducing into the plant genes that encode enzymes that degrade cell wall of fungi and bacteria and do not harm plant cell.

    *   Fungal cell consists of two polymers glucan and chitin that can be broken down by glucanases and chitinases respectively; chitinase gene from *Serralia marcescens* has been successfully introduced into tobacco, tomato, potato, lettuce and sugarbeet to kill phytopathogenic fungus *Rhizoctonia solani*.

    *   Bacterial cell walls are made up of unusual polymers called peptidoglycans which have both protein and carbohydrate components and which can be digested by the enzyme lysozyme.

    By treating various seeds with very dilute solutions of lysozyme the bacteria, which stick to the seed, can be killed. However, lysozyme being a stable enzyme could do considerable harm to the soil microbes that live in the rhizosphere.

4. **Resistance to abiotic stresses**

    *   Important genes involved in the protection against stresses can be isolated and transferred to sensitive plants. A sharp increase in the content of proline is observed during water stress.

    *   Hans Bohnert from University of Arizona thought that many plants respond to drought stress by synthesizing a group of sugars derivatives called polyols (mannitol, sorbitol and so on) that have high levels of polyols may be more resistant to stress.

Biochemists found that cold-hardy plants have more unsaturated fatty acids (linoleic or linolenic) in the phospholipids that form the cellular membrane than cold sensitive plants. The unsaturated fatty acids (fatty acyltransferase) make the membranes more fluid at low temperatures preventing them from solidifying when the temperature drops below 10-12°C.

5. **Molecular breeding**

    *   The discovery of enzymes like restriction endonucleases and Tag DNA polymerase has not only revolutionized research in the field of molecular biology and recombinant DNA technology, but has also helped in speeding up the process of conventional breeding through marker aided selection. Restriction fragment length polymorphisms (RFLPs) have been used to create linkage maps, localizing genes of economic importance to specific chromosomal positions and have thus led to the development of efficient selection strategies for crop improvement programmes. The RFLP approach is being used also for isolation of desired DNA segment and ultimately the desired gene sequence.

Using PCR (polymer chain reaction) technology, random amplified polymorphic DNAs (RAPDs), has been developed which is more efficient and cost effective as compared with RFLP for undertaking marker assisted selection in breeding programmes.

6. **Improved post-harvest crop qualities**

    1. **Extending shelf life of tomatoes:** During ripening softening, conversion of starch to sugar, loss of chlorophyll, synthesis of red pigments and synthesis of aromatic compounds occur. Ripening fruits produce ethylene and this ethylene production starts and accelerates the ripening process. Suppression of ethylene synthesis can be done by using antisense technology in which the gene encoding aminocylopropane carboxylic acid (ACC) synthase or ACC oxidase, the two enzymes involved in the synthesis of ethylene from methionine, has been put in the reverse orientation (shelf-life increase from 1-4 weeks).

        Suppressing cell-wall degrading enzymes, pectin methyl esterase and polygalacturonase enzymes are responsible for softening the tomato cell wall.

    2. **Engineering high-Starch potatoes:** For making chips or frozen fries, the potato should ideally contain about 25% starch by weight. Transferring glucose molecules one at a time from a glucose donor called ADP-glucose to the growing starch molecule makes starch. For starch synthesis ADP-glucose pyrophosphorylase enzyme is necessary and it can be isolated and cloned from a bacterium.

7. **Improving nutritional quality of foods and feeds**

- Monogastric animals such as human, poultry and pigs need more digestible food material for their good nutrition. Cereal proteins are limiting in lysine, tryptophan and threonine, while pulse proteins in sulfur containing amino acids particularly methionine. Modifying genes by encoding for storage proteins; synthetic oligonucleotides that code for lysine, methionine and tryptophan, enzymes insensitive to feedback inhibition and over expression of a methionine rich seed storage protein from a different crop species.

Genes that encode methionine rich (more than 20%) protein found in sunflower, brazil nut can be transferred to other plants such as soybean, canola, alfalfa and clover. Aspartate kinase and dihydropicolinic acid synthase enzymes are responsible for the increase in lysine content in seeds of oil crops. Thioredoxin is a low molecular weight multifunctional disulfide protein acts as reducing disulfide (S-S) groups of storage proteins and enzyme inhibitor proteins. It improves baking and other nutritional quality of foods by inactivating allergens.

8. **Oil modification**

- Plant oils are used in a wide variety of food and non-food applications. The goals of biotechnology have been to produce speciality oils for industrial uses and to remove unwanted fatty acids from oilseed crops.

By using antisense technology to reduce the levels of stearoyl ACP desaturase, the enzyme that converts stearic acid (C_{18}) into oleic acid ($C_{18:1}$), the levels of stearic acid have been increased from 1.6 to 40% in canola seed. Stearic acid is a major constituent in cocoa butter. Castor oil, which contains 90% ricinoleic acid, is very versatile natural oil. The industrial use of castor oil includes the synthesis of nylon, manufacture of lubricants, hydraulic fluids, plastics, cosmetics and other materials. In castor oleic acid.

Enzyme—ricinoleic acid. Gene for C_{12} thioesterase increase C_{12} fatty acid in the new plant species.

9. **Flower colour modification**

- More efforts are being attempted in flower industry to improve flower appearance and post-harvest shelf life. The flower pigments, which are mainly the flavanoids, are synthesized from phenylalanine by a series of enzyme-catalyzed reactions such as cyaniding derivatives give red colour, delphinidin derivatives gives blue colour. By introducing a gene coding for dihydroflavanol 4-reductase (DFR) from maize which catalyses the conversion of dihydrokaempferol (DHK) (colorless) to respective leucopelargonidin, to DHK accumulating petunia lead to a change in flower colour from pale pink to brick red. A gene F 3' 5' H useful for producing delphinidin pigments which gives blue colour to the roses.

10. **Future prospects**

     *   Fundamental studies in molecular biology and biochemistry are
         necessary for further biotechnological advancements. To increase
         the efficiency of plant photosynthesis, much more information on
         the structure, function and regulation of the enzyme nitrogenase
         responsible for catalyzing the reduction of dinitrogen to ammonia
         is available. Since nif genes encoding nitrogenase proteins are
         repressed by oxygen and also nitrogenase proteins are susceptible
         to oxygen, the efficiency of nif genes to cereals seems to be a distant
         possibility. However, the efficiency of nitrogen fixation process can
         be improved through genetic engineering by making Rhizobium
         species tolerant to abiotic stress and by extending the host range of
         efficient rhizobial strains. Using antisense RNA technology can
         develop low lipase activity in rice bran. Similarly low lipoxygenase
         activity in soybean meal can be developed by antisense RNA
         technology. Maize protein deficit in lysine and trptophan can be
         improved by using biotechnology tools. To develop fruits and
         vegetables, which are sweet without sugar or chemical additives by
         introducing, the genes coding for certain plant products, which are
         sugar substitutes. Ex monellin a protein that is found in the fruit of
         an African plant (*Discorephyllum cumminsii* Diels), which is
         approximately 1,00,000 times sweeter than sucrose on a molecular
         basis. Introducing monellin will have another advantage that being
         a protein; it would not have the same metabolic impact as sugar.
         Monellin is a dimmer (A & B) 45 to 50 amino acid residues.

Ripe fruit of *Thaumatococcus danielli* is a tropical plant found in West Africa,
contains a novel protein thaumatin, which is 5000 times sweeter than a
comparable 4% sucrose aqueous solution. This protein consists of 207 amino
acids residues and has a molecular weight of about 22,000. The gene encoding
thaumatin has been cloned and expressed in yeast. This gene may also be
introduced into sugarcane and beet.

Amygdaline is a cyanogenic glucoside present in seeds of cherries, apples,
pears, peaches, apricots, lima bean, white clover, sorghum and cassava due to
the presence of linamarin can be eliminated by manipulating by biotechnological
methods.

RELEVANCE OF BIOTECHNOLOGY TO AGRICULTURE

Biotechnology

*   Biotechnology (biology + technology) can be regarded as the science of
    improving living organism through various technological changes.
    Biotechnology primarily involves biology, biochemistry and engineering

and aims at the manipulation of information flow in living organisms to the requirements of society. Genetic manipulation at the molecular level is something that crosses many disciplines. Through biotechnology "bad" genes can be replaced with "good" ones to help treat genetic diseases of the human being and animals as well as to help the plant crops to defend themselves.

In agriculture biotechnology has already led to a minor revolution in plant and seed production technology giving us the means to tailor crops to meet specific human needs. Biotechnology forms the basis of today's high-tech agriculture.

Exciting Biotechnological possibilities in Agriculture

Some of the most exciting possibilities brought about through biotechnology in agriculture are as follows:

1. **Squeezing higher yield from crops**

   * Through biotechnological research crop yields and improving the way plants use sun's energy during photosynthesis can increase their quality.

2. **Helping crop plants to defend themselves**

   * Biotechnology has enabled scientists to make food, feed and fiber crops more resistant/tolerant to diseases, insect-pests and various physiological stresses, such as extreme temperatures (heat, cold, frost), acidity, alkalinity and salinity, drought conditions. Disease resistance in living organisms is offer conferred by a single gene, which may be relatively easy to move from one plant to another. One way to achieve this goal is through the production of more desirable artificial or synthetic seeds of agricultural crops by direct manipulation of the embryo (somatic embryo genesis).

3. **Creating new crops and their products**

   * It would be possible to give staple cereal food crops like wheat, rice and maize, the ability to make their own nitrogen rich fertilizers, which would entail them to use solar energy to make ammonia directly from the air.

Biotechnology can help to create new hardy crop plants, capable of thriving in acid, alkaline and saline soils and withstanding longer periods of drought.

4. **Genetic diversification of agriculture**

   * It would be possible to engineer crop plants capable of producing medicinal compounds, natural food additives, favours and fragrances. Development of such crops will enable farmers to

diversify crops. The farmers can be encouraged to grow trans-genic crops by building green houses and harvesting drug-producing plants for pharmaceutical companies. Producers can thus switch from the traditional high-volume, low-value crops (grains) to newer low-volume, to high-value crops.

5. **Improved animal productivity**

   • Biotechnology has already made it possible to identify and isolate the genes controlling growth in the unusually large cattle and transfer them to cattle embryos, thus saving considerable time to selectively breed bigger cows. This can be achieved by better understanding of growth regulating genes for the enhancement of growth rates and lean meat content.

It would also be possible to produce protein-enriched milk by bolstering the genes casein producing ability to fetch higher price for milk and its products. It would thus be possible to manipulate animal effectively by deriving higher productivity by less input.

6. **Extension of shelf life of agricultural products**

   • Through biotechnology, it is possible to extend shelf life of perishable agricultural products, such as fruits, vegetables and animal products. For example genetic manipulation of the microorganisms found in meat has enabled to extend shelf life of red meats vacuum packed in modified atmosphere containers at the university of Alberta, Canada.

7. **Engineering trees for better wood quality**

   • It is possible to genetically improve forest trees for higher growth rates, better wood quality as well as development of secondary chemical products of pharmaceutical and medicinal value. Engineering forest trees suited to marginal environments will make it possible to grow forests where none has existed before. Genetic engineering could thus result in the marriage of the concepts of agriculture and forest.

Selected Contribution of Biotechnology to Human Welfare:

1. Medical biotechnology
2. Industrial biotechnology
3. Animal biotechnology
4. Environmental biotechnology
5. Plant biotechnology (Agricultural biotechnology)

A. **Medical Biotechnology**

    1.   Monoclonal antibodies

    2.   DNA probes

    3.   Recombinant vaccines

    4.   Valuable drugs such as insulin, interferon, growth hormones

    5.   Babies of specific sex (by X or Y sperm separation techniques)

    6.   Gene therapy to cure genetic diseases

    7.   Identification of parents/criminals

B. **Industrial Biotechnology**

    1.   Useful compounds such as ethanol, lactic acid, glycerin, citric acid, gluconic acid, acetic acid, acetone, lecithin etc.

    2.   Antibiotics-Penicillin, streptomycin, erythromycin, mitomycin, cycloheximide etc.

    3.   Production of more useful compound by lowering production cost.

    4.   Production of enzymes: α-amylase, proteases, lipases etc.

    5.   Production of single cell proteins (SCP)

    6.   New fuels

    7.   Mineral extractions

    8.   Immobilization of enzymes for repeated industrial use

    9.   Immunotoxins.

   10.   More useful proteins and enzymes

C. **Animal Biotechnology**

    1.   Transgenic animals for increased milk, growth, resistance to diseases etc.

    2.   Hormone-induced super ovulation

    3.   Embryo transfer

D. **Environmental Biotechnology**

    1.   Efficient sewage treatment, deodorization of human excreta

    2.   Degradation of petroleum products and management of oil spills

    3.   Detoxification of wastes and industrial effluents

    4.   Bio-control of plant diseases and insects

E. **Plant Biotechnology**

    1.   Embryo culture production

    2.   Rapid clonal multiplication through meristem culture

3.   Germplasm conservation

4.   Rapid isolation of homozygous lines by anther culture, inter specific hybridization, ovary culture.

5.   Isolation of stable somaclonal variants with improved yield, yield traits/disease resistance/resistance to cold, herbicides, metal toxicity, salt and other abiotic stresses

6.   Gene transfer for beneficial use to the human

7.   Molecular markers e.g. RFLPs and RAPDS for linkage mapping and mapping of quantitative traits loci.

In agriculture, rapid and economic clonal multiplication of fruit and forest trees, production of virus free stocks of clonal cross, creation of novel genetic variations through somaclonal variations and transfer of novel and highly valuable genes (e.g., for disease and insect resistance) through genetic engineering have opened up exciting possibilities in crop production, protection and improvement.

Recombinant DNA Technology : A recombinant DNA molecule is a vector (e.g. a plasmid, phage or virus) into which the desired DNA fragment has been inserted to enable its cloning in an appropriate host.

Chimaeric gene means a gene from one organism joined to regulatory sequences from another organism.

Gene and gene function: Transcription, Translation, Termination stapes occur in this technology.

Gene transmission : Smiconservative replication of DNA ensures transmission of genes from parents to progeny without change (Spontaneous mutation 14^{-4} to 10^{-7} per gene/generation). Transformation of DNA from cell to cell directly. Transduction means transformation of necessary genetic information from viruses cell to another cell. Conjugation means sexual transmission process.

Genetic Engineering of Crop Plants

Biotechnology involves the use of molecular genetic tools to give the economically important systems (crop plants and animals) new characteristics that cannot be achieved through the conventional breeding techniques. To put it simple words in genetic engineering we take pieces of DNA (deoxyribonucleic acid) from here and there and put them together to produce something better (recombinant DNA technology) than what is found in nature.

The 19th century monk, Gregor Mendel, through breeding experiments with pea plants, laid the early foundations of genetics. He found that plants contain factors, which contribute to the inheritance of specific characteristics. Later scientists found these factors to be genes, which are contained in the chromosomes of every cell. In the 1940s a Canadian scientist Dr. Oswald Avery discovered that genes were made of deoxyribonucleic acid, a long thin string of chemicals. In 1953 at Cambridge University, Dr. James Watson and Dr. Francis Crick found that DNA consisted of two inter twisted strands, each composed of chains of four different chemical basis called adenine (A), guanine (G), cytosine (C) and thymine (T). This discovery has paved the way for recombing or engineering DNA to suite human purposes.

Researchers during the early 1970s developed the recombinant DNA technology required to manipulate and transfer genes from one cell to another. They learned now to use a variety of enzymes to cut genes apart and splice them back together. Today we can take a gene from just about any organism, study it, understand it, modify it, make more of it, return it to its original host or transfer it to cells in completely different organisms.

By the end of the 1970s biotechnology was becoming a major business as the scientists, aware of the commercial potential of this technology, began setting up companies. Existing drug and chemical companies such as Monsanto, Biotechnica International and Eli Lilly, began spending enormous sums on biotechnological research, forging their links with university laboratories. To date their greatest successes have occurred with bacteria. These simple single-celled organisms contain plasmids, small loops of self-replicating DNA, which float about in the cell and are ideal for the insertion of new genes. In the late 1970s Genentech isolated the gene for human insulin inserted it into an *Escherichia coli* bacterium and left the altered organism in a fermentation tank to maturity. As the bacterium multiplied it mass produced human insulin, which was purified and sold under the brand, name Humulin.

Bacteria have also been turned into industrial and agricultural products, capable of among other things, digesting crude oil or fertilizing plants. Dr. Aladar Szalay at the University of Alberta, Canada is currently attempting to develop multi-purpose microbes by transferring desirous genes onto already useful bacteria. It may be thus possible to give fertilizing bacteria the ability to kill plant-threating microbes like fungi and nematodes.

Plants and higher animals are more difficult to engineer genetically, because their cells lack plasmids. Hence, more sophisticated methods are needed to insert new genetic material into them. The new genes must also be properly controlled to switch on and off at the right time and place. For example, an insect-repelling gene should produce its toxin only when the insect is in season and only in those plant parts that are likely to be attacked. Although we can put only gene into only plant, gene expression varies from organ to organ. Not all genes are active in every cell. We must therefore learn how to control the signals that turn genes on and off in order to engineer them intelligently. Identifying and isolating "switches" and hooking them to appropriate genes are a major task ahead for the biotechnological researchers.

Virtually any known gene can be chemically assembled in the laboratory with a computerized DNA synthesizer. The switch-gene combination is chemically connected to marker genes (luciferase) plus another gene resistant to particular drug. This is all accomplished in a test tube (*in vitro*) by a variety of enzymes that cut paste DNA into the desired sequence. Once the genetic material has been "designed" it is inserted into bacteria, which quickly produce, copies of the stuff thus giving the scientist plenty of material with which to experiment. Next the genetic material is transferred into selected plant cells, which can be done in one of several ways. The cell membranes must be opened to allow the foreign DNA inside where it is incorporated into the chromosomes and passed on to subsequent generations of cells.

The success of gene transfer can be ascertained by putting the petridish of cells into the chamber of a computerized "lowlight video image analyzing system" where the cells are scanned by an extremely sensitive camera capable of detecting the light emitted by the marker luciferase genes. Plant cells, which have taken up the foreign luciferase containing DNA will give off light and show up clearly on the computer screen connected to the photo chamber. The cells are placed into a nutrient medium where they develop into a callus a cluster of undifferentiated cells resembling colored sugar crystals. The callus is placed in another medium containing hormones that encourage leaves and roots to grow. Finally the plant let is potted and grow to maturity. Every cell in the "regenerated" plant contains a copy of the transferred gene. These plants are then observed for the new gene's effect. Apart from genetic engineering, several other molecular marker techniques such as Restriction Fragment Length Polymorphism (RFLP), Random Amplified Polymorphic DNA (RAPD) are being used successfully in agriculture, in addition to gene transfer, tissue culture and hormonal bio-regulation of crops composition. Using these techniques scientists at ICRISAT are trying to improve crop plants like groundnut by transferring genes from wild *Arachis* spp. into the cultivated ones.

Steps in Gene Cloning

1. Identification and isolation of the desired gene or DNA fragment to be cloned.

2. Insertion of the isolated gene in a suitable vector.

3. Introduction of this vector into a suitable organism/cell called host (transformation).

4. Selection of the transformed host cells; and

5. Multiplication/expression/integration followed by expression of the introduced gene in the host.

Isolation of the desired gene : The identification and isolation of the desired gene or DNA fragment called DNA insert to be cloned is a critical step in gene cloning.

This can be obtained from

1. cDNA libraries, 2. Genomic library 3. Chemical (or enzymatic) synthesis and 4. Amplification through polymerase chain reaction (PCR).

Preparation of cDNA

cDNA is the copy or complementary DNA produced by using mRNA (usually) as a template. DNA copy of an RNA molecule is produced by the enzyme reverse transcriptase (RNA-dependent DNA polymerase; discovered by Temin and Baltimore in 1970) from avian mycloblastosis virus (AMV). This enzyme performs similar reactions as DNA polymerase and has an absolute requirement for a primer with a free 3′ –OH.

Gene Amplification through Polymerase Chain Reaction

The polymerase chain reaction (PCR) technique, developed by Kary Mullis in 1985 is extremely powerful. It generates microgram (mg) quantities of DNA copies (upto billion copies) of the desired DNA (or RNA) segment, present even as   single copy in the initial preparation, in a matter of few hours.

The PCR is carried out in vitro. It utilizes 1. A DNA preparation containing the desired segment to be amplified. 2. Two nucleotide primers (about 20 bases long), specific, i.e. complementary to the two 3′ borders (the sequences present at the 3′ ends of the two strands) of the desired segment. 3. The four-deoxynucleoside triphosphates viz., TTP (thymidine triphosphate), dCTP (deoxycyctidine triphosphate), dATP (deoxyadenosine triphosphate) and dGTP (deoxyguanosine triphosphate) and a heat stable DNA polymerase, e.g., Tag (isolated from bacterium the *Thermus acquaticus*), Pfu (from *Pyrococcus furiosus*) and Vent (from *Thermococcus litoralis*) polymerases. Pfu and Vent polymerases are more efficient than the Tag polymerase.

Multiplication, expression and integration of the DNA insert in host genome

Once the clone containing the desired DNA insert is identified, it is multiplied in *E. coli* to obtain sufficient number of copies to be used in one or more of the following ways.

1. It can be used for a structural analysis of the insert, e.g., DNA sequencing, chromosome walking etc.

2. It may be introduced into a bacterium like *B. subtilis* for production of the protein encoded by the insert sine this host secretes proteins into the medium, which allows easy purification.

3. It can be introduced into a eukaryotic host, e.g., yeast, animal cells, plants etc. either to investigate the function of the insert or

4. To integrate it into the host genome to achieve one of many diverse objectives.

Southern hybridization : The name of this technique is derived from the name of its inventor E.M. Southern and the DNA-DNA hybridization that forms its basis. It is also called Southern blotting since the procedure for transfer of DNA from the get to the nitrocellulose filter resembles blotting. This technique has since been extended to the analysis of RNA (northern blotting) and proteins (western blotting); these names are only jargon terms.

Dot blot technique : This technique is used to detect the presence of a given sequence of DNA/RNA in the non-fractionated (not subjected to gel electrophoresis) DNA.

Northern hybridization : RNAs are separated by gel electrophoresis; the RNA bands are transferred onto a suitable membrane, e.g., diazobenzyloxymethyl (DBM) paper or nylon membranes and immobilized; the bands are hybridized with radioactive single-stranded DNA by autoradiography. It is an extension of the Southern blotting technique.

Southern blotting technique	Northern blotting technique
DNA is separated by gel electrophoresis	RNAs are separated by gel electrophoresis
DNA has to be denatured before blotting	Not needed in this protocol
Nitrocellulose membrane is used in this system	Diazobenzyloxymethyl (DBM) paper is used in this system
Hybridization with the probe produces DNA-DNA hybrid molecules	RNA : DNA molecules produces in this system

Recently developed nylon membranes have superceded the use of DBM paper as they are robust, reusable and bind (by cross linking) to RNA on a brief exposure to UV light.

Northern hybridization is useful in the identification and separation of the RNA that is complementary to a specific DNA probe; this is a sensitive test for the detection of transcription of a DNA sequence that is used as probe.

Western blotting : Proteins are electrophoresed in polyacrylamide gel transferred onto a nitrocellulose or nylon membrane (to which they bind strongly), and the protein bands are detected by their specific interaction with antibodies, lectins or some other compounds.

The specific protein bands are identified in a variety of ways: Antibodies are the most commonly used as probes for detecting specific antigens. Lectins are used as probes for the identification of glycoproteins. These probes may themselves be radioactive or a radioactive molecule may be tagged to them. Often the identification process is based on a "Sandwich" reaction.

Probes : Probes are small (15-30 bases long) nucleotide sequences used to detect the presence of complementary sequences in nucleic acid samples. This is achieved by permitting the probes to base pair with the sample nucleic acids and then identifying the samples that show base pairing with the probes, i.e., hybridization.

Both DNA and RNA are used as probes. Single-stranded DNA probes are more convenient and preferable, but denatured double stranded DNA molecules can also be used.

Nick translation : This is the oldest method of nucleic acid labeling and is still the most commonly used. This technique is quite flexible with respect to probe size, specific activity and concentration; it is particularly suited for the production of large quantities of probes for use in multiple hybridization reactions and/or where a high probe concentration is required.

Enzyme-linked immunosorbent assay [ELISA] : An antibody (Ab) reacts with the concerned antigen (Ag) in a highly specific manner (i.e., an antibody reacts with that determinant or region of an antigen for which it is specific) to produce an Ag-Ab complex. When soluble proteins react with an antibody, the Ag-Ab complex forms a precipitate, while incase of particulate antigens the Ag-Ab complex agglutinates. In either case, either the amount of Ag-Ab complex formed or the rate of its formation is used to determine either quantity of the antigen or that of the antibody involved in the interaction. The various assays used for the following purposes:

Precipitation reaction, the ouchterlony assay, the mancini assay, immunoelectrophoresis, western blotting, rocket electrophoresis, agglutination reactions, labeled antibody techniques, radioimmune assay (RIA), enzyme-linked immuno-sorbent assay, fluorescent labels, electron dense labels, non specific binding to immunoglobulin and flow cytometry.

In situ **hybridization :** In situ hybridization has been used to establish the location of sat-DNA in chromosomes. For this purpose, radioactive copies of sat-DNA or its complementary RNA (using sat-DNA as template) are prepared. Chromosomes in squash preparations are specially pretreated to expose and denature their DNA without affecting their structural integrity. These chromosomes are then loaded with the radioactive single-stranded sat-DNA or its complementary RNA-after an appropriate interval, the squash preparations are washed to remove the nonhybridized radioactive DNA (or RNA) probe and the location of radioactivity in the chromosomes is determined through radio autographic technique.

In situ or cytological hybridization is also used to locate specific genes in chromosomes, especially in giant chromosomes. For this purpose, a radioactive clone representing a gene, most often labeled cDNA copies of the mRNA produced by the gene, is used as probe. Colony hybridization is also a form of Situ hybridization. This technique is also useful in disease diagnosis, particularly for the detection of viruses in tissues and cells.

Cloning : Cells derived from a single cell through mitosis constitute a clone and the process of obtaining clones is called cloning. (A sexual progeny of a single individual make up a clone). In simple term, cloning consists of trypsinisation of a monolayer culture to prepare a cell suspension, 3-4 dilution steps to achieve a suitable cell density (10-200 cells/ml), and seeding in petri dishes or flasks or multi-well dishes. The culture vessels are incubated for 1-3 weeks with a medium change after 1 wee; by this time colonies will develop.

Cloning is used to:

1. Obtain homogeneous cell lines from heterogeneous cell cultures.

2. To isolate biochemical mutants

3. Cell strains with marker chromosomes and

4. To develop hybridoma clones.

Cloning is generally applied to continuous cell lines, but often their clones become considerably heterogeneous by the time they are sufficiently multiplied for use. The problem with finite cell lines is that of life span; by the time the clone is sufficiently multiplied, the cells may be approaching senescence.

DNA Fingerprinting : DNA fingerprinting or DNA profiling is generally used for the identification of criminals from blood strains, semen etc. and for establishing parentage in cases of dispute. The data from this approach are extremely reliable as compared to the conventional analysis of serum proteins and erythrocyte antigens and proteins. DNA fingerprint of an individual is essentially a Southern blot of this DNA digested with an endonuclease and probed with a radioactive DNA probe.

Molecular Markers : Isozymes (electrophoretic variants of enzymes) and DNA sequences are used as molecular markers in chromosome mapping. Therefore, for all practical purposes, a molecular marker may be defined as a DNA sequence used for chromosome mapping, as it can be located at a specific site in a chromosome. A molecular marker may be either anonymous or defined. An anonymous marker is a cloned random DNA fragment whose function or specific features are not known. Defined marker may contain a gene or some other specific feature e.g. Restriction sites for rare cutting restriction enzymes etc.

1. Estriction fragment length polymorphism (RFLP)

2. Random amplified polymorphic DNAs (RAPD)

3. Variable number of tandem repeats (VNTRs) DNA

    a. Minisatellite DNAs

    b. Microsatellite DNAs

4. CPG islands: About 1% of the human chromosomal DNA is stably unmethylated; these regions are called CPG islands since they contain more than 50% of C + G.

5. Isozymes

6. Short tandem repeat (STR) DNA.

A comparison between RFLP and RAPD markers for genome mapping in plants:

Feature	RFLP	RAPD
Inheritance pattern	Codominant	Dominant
Detection of multiple alleles of a marker	Yes	No
Quality of DNA needed for study	Pure	Crude
Amount of DNA needed	2-10 mg	>10 ng
Radio isotopes	Must be used (in probes)	Not used
Restriction enzymes	Must be used	Not used
Type of probe used	Species specific probes, generally low copy genomic or DNA	Random base sequence 9-12 base nucleotides
Time required	About 5 times more than RAPDs	0.20 % of that for RFLPs

Biochemical Production by Biotechnology

Plants are the source of a large variety of biochemicals that are metabolites of both primary and secondary metabolism. But secondary metabolites are of much greater interest since they have impressive biological activities like antimicrobial, antibiotic, insecticidal, molluscidal, hormonal properties and valuable pharmacological and pharmaceutical activities and many are used as flavours, fragrances, colours etc.

Some of the Biochemicals Obtained from Plants

Group of chemical	Examples
Alkaloids	Morphine, codeine, quinine, nicotine, cocaine, hyoscyamine, lysergic acid etc.
Terpenoids	Menthol, camphor, carotenoid pigments, polyterpenes (e.g., rubber) etc.
Phenylpropanoids	Anthocyanins, coumarines, flavonoids, isoflavonoids, stilbenes, tannins etc.
Quinones	Anthraquinones, benzoquinones, naphthoquinones
Steroids	Diosgenin, sterols, ferruginol etc.

Products generated from genetically engineered microbes (GEMS). The products are either in current therapeutic use or in advanced stages of development.

Product	GEM	Application
Insulin	E. coli & yeast	Diabetes
Human growth hormone	E. coli	Dwarfism
Interferons	E. coli	Viral diseases, cancer, AIDS
Interleukins	E. coli	Various cancers
Hepatitis-B surface antigen	Yeast	Vaccine against hepatitis-B
Streptokinase	E. coli	Thrombolysis
Epidermal growth factor	E. coli	Wound and burn healing
Granulocyte macrophage colony stimulating factor	E. coli	Cancer, AIDS, Bone marrow transplantation
Bovine growth hormone	E. coli	Increased milk yield
Tumor necrosis factor	E. coli	Sepsis, Cancer

Some restriction endonucleases, the organisms in which they naturally occur (source) :

Restriction /endonuclease	Source (organism & strain)	Recognition sequence
AvaI	Anabaena variabilis (ATCC 27892)	C/Py CGPuGGpuGC Py/C
AluI	Arthrobacter luteus	AG/CT, TC/GA
BamHI	Bacillus amyloliquefaciens H	G/G AT CC,CCTA G/G
ECOR I	Escherichia Coli Ry13	G/AA TTC, CTT AA/G
ECOR II	E. Coli R245	/CCA(T) GG, GGT(A) CC/
Bgl II	Bacillus globigli	A/G ATCTTCTAG/A
Hind II	Haemophilus influenzae Rd	GT Py/Pu ACCA Pu/Py TG
Hind III	Haemophilus influenzae Rd	A/A GCTTTCG A/A
Hind II	H. influenzae P1	G/G CC, CC G/G
Hpa I	H. Parainfluenzae	GTT/AAC, CAA/TTG
Hpa II	H. parainfluenzae	C/C GG, GG C/C
Hinf1	H. influenzae Rf	G/A NTC, CTNA/G
N/a III	Neisseria lactamica	CATG/, /GTAC
Pst I	Providencia stuartii	CTGCA/G, G/ACGTC
Sau 3A	Staphylococcus aureus 3A	/GATC, CTAG/
Taq I	Thermus aquaticus YTI	T/C GA, AGC/T

Different effects of plant growth regulators in plant tissue culture systems

Plant growth regulators	Short forms	Main effects in culture
Auxins	IAA, IBA, NAA, 2,4-D; 2,4,5-T, Picloram, Dicamba, CPA	Adventitious root formation (at high concentration) Adventitious shoot formation (at low concentration) Induction of somatic embryos (particularly 2,4-D)

Contd...

Plant growth regulators	Short forms	Main effects in culture
		Cell division
		Differentiation of vascular tissue
		Callus formation and growth
		Inhibition of outgrowth of axillary buds
		Inhibition of root growth
Cytokinins	Zn, ZnR, 2-ip, IPA,	Stimulation of shoot initiation/bud formation
		Inhibition
	BAP, Kn, TDZ, CPPU	of root formation
		Cell division
		Callus formation and growth
		Stimulation of outgrowth of axillary buds
		Promotion of rejuvenation of mature shoots
		Inhibition of shoot elongation
		Inhibition of leaf/shoot senescence
		Promotion of some stages of root development
		Stimulation of the dark-germination of light-development seeds.
Gibberellins	GA_1, GA_3, GA_4, GA_7	Promotion of internodes elongation
		Loss of dormancy in seed, somatic embryos, apical buds and bulbs
		Inhibition of adventitious root formation
		Synthesis of inhibitors which promote tuber, corm and bulb formation
		Regulation of the transition from juvenile to adult phases
		Synthesis of inhibitors which facilitate acclimatization
Abscisic acid	-	Maturation of somatic embryos
		Promotion of desiccation tolerance of the somatic embryos
		Promotion of the accumulation of storage protein during embryogenesis
		Inhibition of precocious germination of somatic embryos
		Bulb and tuber formation
		Promotion of the development of dormancy
		Promotion of senescenceInhibition of elongation
Ethylene	-	Senescence of leaves
		Promotion or inhibition of adventitious regeneration depending upon the species and phase of culture
		Breaking of seed and bud dormancy in some species
		Inhibition of adventitious roots and root hairs
Polymines	Putrescine Spermidine Spermine	Promotion of adventitious root formationPromotion of shoot formation Promotion of somatic embryogenesis
Jasmonic acid	-	Promotion of tuber and bulb formation
		Enhancement of meristem formation
		Stimulation of root formation

Contd...

Plant growth regulators	Short forms	Main effects in culture
		Promotion of tissue differentiation
		Inhibition of root length growth
		Breaking of seed dormancy
		Promotion of pigment formation
Brassino-steroids	-	Promotion of shoot elongation
		Inhibition of root growth and development
		Enhancement of xylem differentiation
		Promotion of germination
Salicylic acid	-	Inhibition of seed germination
		Blocking of the wound response
		Promotion of bud formationInduction of flowering

Give the list of common compounds generally used for the preparation of basal media?

Compound used	Molecular weight
Major salts	
$CaCl_2.2H_2O$	147.02
$Ca(NO_3)_2.4H_2O$	236.15
KH_2PO_4	136.09
KNO_3	101.10
$MgSO_4.7H_2O$	246.50
NH_4NO_3	80.09
NH_4Cl	53.49
$(NH_4)_2SO_4$	132.14
K_2HPO_4	174.18
H_3BO_3	61.84
Minor salts	
$CoCl_2.6H_2O$	237.93
$CuSO_4.5H_2O$	249.68
$Na_2 EDTA.2H_2O$	372.20
$FeSO_4.7H_2O$	278.00
KCl	74.56
KI	166.01
$MnSO_4.4H_2O$	223.09
$Na_2MoO_4.2H_2O$	241.95
$ZnSO_4.7H_2O$	287.55
Vitamins and amino acids	
Biotin	244.32
Calcium pantothenate	476.53
Folic acid	441.41
Pantothenic acid	219.24

Contd...

Compound used	Molecular weight
r-Aminobenzoic acid	137.13
L-Ascorbic acid	176.12
Nicotinic acid	123.11
Riboflavin	376.36
Thiamin hydrochloride	337.28
Pyridoxine hydrochloride	205.64
Glycine	75.07
Myoinositol	180.16
Plant growth regulators	
Adenine	135.13
Adenine sulphate	368.34
2,4-D	221.04
NAA	186.21
IBA	203.24
IAA	175.19
Kinetin	215.22
2-ip	203.25
BAP	225.26
TDZ	220.25

Different secondary metabolites produced by different plants

Compound	Source of plant and parts	Activity
Monoterpene		
Pyrethyroids	Chrysanthemum, leaves and flowers	Insecticidal
Limonene, myrcene	Pine, needles, twigs and trunk	Toxic to insects
Essential oils (flavour and fragrance)		Insect repellant
(a) Peppermint oil (Menthol)	Mentha, glandular hairs	
(b) Lemon oil (limonene)	Lemon, glandular hair	
(c) Lavendula		
(d) Eucalyptus oil	Lavendula angustifolia	Eucalyptus
Gossypol cotton	Pigment gland	Against insects, fungus, bacteria
Artemisinin	*Artemisia annua*	Against malaria, cerebral malaria
Diterpene		
Taxol	*Taxus wallichiana*, needles, barks	Novel anti-cancer drug for breast and ovarian cancer
Resin	*Hymenaea courbaril*	As glue
Forskolin	*Coleus forskolhii*	Anti-hypertension, anti-glucoma

Contd...

Compound	Source of plant and parts	Activity
Triterpene (diverse compounds)		
Steriods (Solasodine)	*Solanum nigram*	Steroidal drug
Limonoids	Citrus fruit	Bitter substance, helps in digestion
Azadirachtin	Neem tree	Most efficient deterrent to insect feeding
Cardenolides with attached sugars (gly cosides)Digitoxin Bufadinolide	Digitalis purpurea (Fox glove)*Urgibea indica*	Bitter in taste, toxic to higher animals, in humans they act positively on heart musclesTreatment of heart disease
Saponins	Dioscorea	Anti-fertility compound
Polyterpene		
Rubber (milky latex)	*Hevae* Sp. *Manilkara-in laticifers*	Wound healing, defense
Phenolics		
Tannins	Tea, apple, blackberry, red wine	General toxin, reduces growth & survival of herbivores, to preserve animal skin
Lignins	*Podophyllum hexandrum*	Physical deterrant to feeding, cytostatic
Flavonoids Anthocyanins	Red, pink, purple, blue, colours in plant cells	Visual and olfactory attractants
Alkaloids		
Nicotine	Tobacco	Precursor of vit. B. Stimulant of the CNS, physiologically addicting drug
Opium, morphine (heroin), codeine, papaverine	Poppy	Important medicinal compound
Cocaine	Coca	Against alcoholism & depression
Caffeine	Coffee, tea, cocoa	CNS stimulant, mild diuretic, effect on metabolic rate, used to produce chocolate and colas
Berberine	*Coptis*, roots	
Ephedrine	*Ephedra*, shoots	
Cyanogenic glycosides	Cassava tubers	Source of hydrogen cyanide, a poisonous gas
Colchicine	*Colchicum, Gloriossa*	Antimitotic/cytostatic

Clone

The conventional dictionary definition of clone provides several possible answers to the question.

A clone can be:

1. A group of genetically identical individuals descended from the same parent by asexual reproduction. Many plants show this by producing suckers, tubers or bulbs to colonise the area around the parent.

2. A group of DNA molecules produced from an original length of DNA sequences produced by a bacterium or a virus using molecular biology techniques. This is what is often called molecular cloning or DNA cloning or simply cloning.

3. A group genetically identical produced by mitotic division from an original cell. This is where the cell creates a new set of chromosomes and splits into two daughter cells. This is how replacement cells are produced in your body when the old ones wear out.

What are the advantages and disadvantages of using *E. coli* as a host of gene cloning?

Advantages

1. Genetics and biochemistry are well understood
2. Plasmids are stable
3. Can accept many types of vector
4. Many strains exist with useful mutations
5. Favours high exist yield of vector DNA
6. High yield of protein

Disadvantages

1. Not a GRAS organism
2. No capacity for intron splicing
3. Limited secretion of proteins into the culture medium
4. Produces endotoxins as part of the outer layer of cell wall
5. Proteins are not glycosylated
6. Does not synthesise disulphydryl bonds
7. Proteins might be insoluble
8. Proteins might be unstable

List of genetically modified crops with their specific characteristics

Crop	Character
Tomato	Modified ripening, Delayed ripening
Soya beans	Glyphosate tolerance, High oleic acid content of oil
Potato	Insect resistance
Cotton	Bromoxynil tolerance, Insect resistance, Glyphosate tolerance, Sulphonylurea tolerance, Herbicide tolerance
Squash	Virus resistance
Oilseed rape	Glyphosate tolerance, High laurate oil
Oilseed	Glufosinate tolerance
Maize	Insect resistance, Male sterile, Glufosinate tolerance, Glyphosate tolerance, Herbicide tolerance.
Chicory	Male sterile
Rice	Vitamin A

5

REASONING

Why biotechnology is very important in relation to human being, animals, microorganisms and plants too?

What is the biotechnological contribution related to human welfare?

The most important contribution of biotechnology related to human welfare is given in following table in detail.

S. No.	Product	Remarks
A. Plant Biotechnology		
1.	Embryo culture to rescue otherwise in viable hybrids to recover haploid plants from interspecific hybrids, micro propagation of orchids etc.	The first two applications are the most remarkable.
2.	Rapid clonal multiplication through meristem culture such as many fruit and forest trees like teak.	Very high rates of multiplication, conventional rates very low.
3.	Recovery of virus and other pathogen free stocks of clonal crops; meristem culture is generally combined with thermotherapy/cryotherapy.	Very useful in clonal crops; particularly for Germplasm exchange.
4.	Germplasm conservation through storage in liquid nitrogen −196°C cryo-preservation or through slow growth.	Particularly useful in clonal crops, especially in those producing tubers, storage roots etc.
5.	Rapid isolation of homozygous lines by chromosome doubling of haploids produced through anther culture/interspecific hybridization/ovary culture.	Very successful in variety development in China such as rice and wheat.
6.	Isolation of stable somaclonal variants with improved yield/yield traits/disease resistance/resistance to cold, herbicides, metal toxicity, salt and other abiotic stresses.	Many examples of successful isolation; may variations are stable and heritable; often due to gene mutations, which may sometimes be novel.
7.	Gene transfers for insect resistance, protection against viruses, herbicide resistance, storage protein improvement etc.	Mainly using the Ti plasmid of *Agrobacterium*; also through particle gun, free DNA uptake; revolutionary development in crop improvement.
8.	Molecular markers such as RFLPs and RAPDs for linkage mapping and mapping of quantitative trait loci.	A powerful too for indirect selection for quantitative traits; several other important applications.

Contd...

S. No.	Product	Remarks
B. Animal Biotechnology		
1.	Test tube babies in humans; involves *in vitro* fertilization and embryo transfer.	Couples suffering from infertility can be having babies.
2.	Hormone induced super ovulation and/or embryo splitting in farm animals; involving embryo transfer and in many cases, *in vitro* fertilization.	For rapid multiplication of animals of superior genotype.
3.	Production of transgenic animals for increased milk, growth rate, resistance to diseases and production of some valuable proteins in milk/urine/blood etc.	Transgenic mice, pigs, chicken, rabbits, cattle, sheep, fish produced.
C. Medical Biotechnology		
1.	Monoclonal antibodies used for disease diagnosis such as venereal diseases, hepatitis B and other viral diseases, cancer etc.	Produced by hybridoma technology
2.	DNA probes used for disease diagnosis such as kal-azar, sleeping sickness, malaria etc.	Produced by genetically engineered microbes.
3.	Recombinant vaccines clear, safer such as human hepatitis B virus, *E. coli* vaccines for pigs, rabies virus etc.	Produced by genetically engineered microbes.
4.	Valuable drugs like insulin, human interferon, human and bovine growth hormones etc.	Produced by genetically engineered bacteria.
5.	Gene therapy to cure genetic diseases such as Huntington's chorea, cystic fibrosis.	Techniques in advanced stages of development.
6.	Babies of specified sex, artificial insemination with X or Y carrying sperms prepared by sperm separation techniques.	It is feared that this may unfavorably change the sex ratio in the population.
7.	Identification of parents/criminals using DNA or autoantibody fingerprinting.	Very accurate and reliable; from even blood or semen stains, hair roots etc.
D. Industrial Biotechnology		
1.	Production of useful compounds such as ethanol, lactic acid, glycerine, citric acid, gluconic acid, acetone etc.	Produced by microorganisms mainly bacteria, from less useful substrate.
2.	Production of antibiotics such as penicillin, streptomycin, erythromycin, mitomycin, cycloheximide etc.	Produced by fungi, bacteria and actinoycetes as secondary metabolites.
3.	Transformation of less useful and cheaper compounds into more useful and valuable ones such as steroid hormones from sterols, sorbose from sorbitol etc.	Generally by microorganisms or immobilized enzymes as secondary metabolites.

Contd...

S. No.	Product	Remarks
4.	Production of enzymes such as a-amylase, proteases, lipases etc.	From fungi, bacteria etc. for use in detergent, textile, leather, dairy industries and in medicines.
5.	Single cell proteins from bacteria, yeasts, fungi or algae for human food and animal feed as a supplements.	Single cell proteins are the total microbial biomass freed from toxins, contaminants, if any.
6.	Fuel mainly ethanol, sometimes biogas production from cheap, less useful and abundant substrates such as sugarcane bagasse, wood etc.	Produced through fermentation by microorganisms. Cowdungbased biogas being popularized in India.
7.	Mineral extraction through leaching from low grade ores such as copper, uranium etc.	Due to action of microbes, mainly bacteria.
8.	Immobilization of enzymes for their repeated industrial application.	More attractive than the use of whole microorganisms.
9.	Protein/enzyme engineering to change the primary structure of existing proteins/ enzymes to make them more efficient, change their substrate specificity such as successes with T4 lysozyme, trypsin, subtilisin, lactate dehydrogenase etc.	Extensive use of computers for generating models of protein molecules. It is hoped to change RuBisCo so as to minimize its affinity for O_2.
10.	Production of immunotoxins by joining a natural toxin with a specific antibody.	These destroy specific cell types; may provide a potent treatment for cancer.
E. Environmental Biotechnology		
1.	Efficient sewage treatment, deodorization of human excreta.	Efficient strains of microorganisms developed
2.	Degradation of petroleum and management of oil spills	A strain of *Pseudomonas putida*.
3.	Detoxification of wastes and industrial effluents	Genetically engineered microbes.
4.	Biocontrol of plant diseases and insect pests by using viruses, bacteria, amoebae fungi etc.	Environment friendly; avoids the use of pesticides which cause pollution.

Secondary metabolites produced on large scale using biotechnological tool

Many plants are good source of a large variety of biochemicals, which are metabolites of both primary and secondary metabolism. The secondary metabolites are of much greater interest since they have impressive biological activities like antimicrobial, antibiotic, insecticidal, molluscidal, hormonal properties, and valuable pharmacological and pharmaceutical activities, and many are used as flavours, fragrances, colours etc.

List of secondary metabolites produced on large scale using biotechnology.

Sr. No.	Group of compound	Examples
1.	Alkaloids	Morphine, codeine, quanine, nicotine, cocaine, hyoscyamine, lysergic acid etc.
2.	Terpenoids	Menthol, camphor, carotenoid pigments, poyterpenes etc.
3.	Phenylpropanoids	Anthocyanins, coumarins, flavonoids, isoflavonoids, stilbenes, tannins etc.
4.	Quinones	Anthraquinones, benzoquinones, naphthoquinones etc.
5.	Steroids	Diosgenin, sterols, ferruginol etc.

Higher plants are the rich source of a large number of pharmaceutically important biochemicals; about 25% of the prescribed medicines are solely derived from plants. Many of these pharmaceutical compounds have complex structures, which makes their chemical synthesis economically unattractive. But some compounds yield is very low from plant tissues prevents their commercial application. In this case the biotechnology can make drastic change in the production of such compounds from plants.

Some of the pharmaceutical biochemicals obtained from plants.

Sr. No.	Compound	Plant species	Medicinal value
1.	Shikonin	*Lithospermum erythrorhizon*	Antiseptic; used as dye for silk and cosmetics
2.	Berberine	*Coptis japonica*	Antibacterial, anti-inflammatory
3.	Codeine	*Papaver somniferum*	Analgesic
4.	Diosgenin	*Dioscorea deltoidea*	Antifertility agents
5.	Quinine	*Cinchona*	Antimalarial
6.	Scopolamine	*Datura stramonium*	Antihypertensive
7.	Vincristine	*Catharanthus roseus*	Antileukaemic
8.	Ajmalicin	*Catharanthus roseus*	Antileukaemic
9.	Taxol	*Taxus species*	Breast and ovarian cancer treatment
10.	Artemisin	*Artemisia sp.*	Antimalarial
11.	Trichosanthin and Karasurin	*Trichosanthes sp.*	Cytotoxicity against HIV infected cells, immunosuppressant, induces abortion.

Role of Biotechnology in Fuel Production from Agriculture Field

Ethanol/Alcohol Fuel Production from Agricultural Produce:

Alcohol has assumed very important place in the Country's economy. It is vital raw material for a number of chemicals. It has been a source of large amount of revenue by way of Excise Duty levied by State Government on Alcohol liquors. It has a potentiality as fuel in the form of power alcohol for blending with petrol in the ratio of 20:80. Fermentation alcohol has great demand in countries like Japan, United States, Canada and Sri Lanka etc. The systematic alcohol produced by these countries from Naphtha of Petroleum crude is not useful for beverages. Large quantities of alcohol were exported out of country during last few years. The target of alcohol demand as projected in the perspective plan for Chemical Industry, Department of Chemical and Petrochemicals is 3000 million liters per annum by year 2010.

Ethyl alcohol is an important feedstock for the manufacture of chemicals. These chemicals are primarily the basic carbon based products like Acetic acid, Butanol, Butadiene, Acetic anhydride, Vinyl acetate, PVC etc. (**Figure 1**). Acetic acid and butanol, which are needed in Pharmaceuticals, paints and in many other areas are important industries as they are value added precuts.

Ethylene, ethylene Oxide and Mono-ethylene glycol are also produced from petrochemical route. However, with latest technological development and taking into account the increasing cost of basic petrochemical raw material, it is now possible to produce Ethylene Oxide, Mono-ethylene Glycol etc. starting from ethanol.

In special applications, absolute alcohol with 99.8 to 99.9% ethyl alcohol content is required. Therefore, it is necessary to produce absolute alcohol with 99.9% purity and select an appropriate technology. The characteristics of absolute alcohol are given in the following table.

Characteristics of absolute alcohol

Description	Characteristics of absolute alcohol
Specific gravity at 15.6 ^{0}C	0.7961
Molecular weight	46
Oxygen content	34.70%
Latent vapourization heat	925 KJ/Kg
Lower calorific value	27723 KJ/Kg, 6642 Kcal/Kg
Boiling point	78.30 ^{0}C
Energy per unit and volume	22012 KJ/Kg
Viscosity at 20°C	1.192
Vapour pressure at 20°C	0.058 Atm
Vapour pressure at 40°C	0.177 Atm
Vapour pressure at 60°C	0.463 Atm
Octane number (research) RON	106
Octane number (motor) MON	87
Stoichiometric mixture	8.95:1 Air: Fuel

This purified alcohol is called as extra neutral alcohol. It is also useful for cosmetics and perfumes. Absolute alcohol is water free ethyl alcohol and is generally used for purification of pharmaceutical products. The material shall be a clear, colourless and homogenous liquid, free from suspended matter and consisting essentially of ethanol. The process of producing anhydrous alcohol for use as fuel-ethanol is fairly standardized. The technology is available in India and Industrial scale plants are operating, currently for use in the industrial and pharmaceutical applications.

The process of dehydration of rectified spirit entails distillation of the spirit along with an entrainer like hexane. This entrainer takes with itself water present in the spirit, thus rendering the alcohol anhydrous. This water is than separated from hexane in another distillation column, thus recycling hexane.

Fuel Ethanol as an Oxygenate

Fuel-ethanol could be used in petrol as an oxygenate. They reduce emission of carbon monoxide in the exhaust gases of vehicles, by taking combustion to completion. It is necessary and advisable to reduce emission of carbon monoxide because it is toxic to human beings. Completion of combustion also reduces emission of particulate carbon matter, which could cause respiratory disorders. Oxygenate has "in-built" oxygen molecule which helps in completing combustion in a better manner. Oxygenates are organic compounds having boiling point in the vicinity of the boiling point of petrol. These compounds mix easily and thoroughly with petrol. Other compounds which are commonly used as oxygenates are tetraethyl lead, MTBE (Methyl-tert-butyl ether), ETBE (ethyl tert-butyl ether), methanol etc. These compounds are also having oxygen molecules in them.

Other function of the compounds added as oxygenates is octane enhancer and anti-knocking agent. These compounds improve the octane number of petrol, thus improving its combustion. Tetraethyl lead is an oxygenate which is rich in oxygen. It has been traditionally used as an oxygenate in petrol. However, it emits poisonous and dangerous fumes containing lead, which are suspected to cause cancer. In order to replace tetraethyl lead, other substances are added to petrol like the aromatics fraction from crude petroleum distillation. This fraction containing BTX-benzene, toluene and xylene is added to improve the octane number. However, emissions from such a mixture are poisonous and require a catalytic converter to prevent such emissions. Thus, vehicles using BTX fractions in petrol have to use a catalytic converter on the exhaust of their vehicle. When MTBE is used as oxygenating agent, there is a danger of it contaminating surface water making it unsuitable for use. In order to get the required content of oxygen, various oxygenates have to be added in different proportion to petrol, based on their content of oxygen.

Process of Manufacturing Dehydrated fuel

Absolute alcohol is an important product required by industry. It is 100% alcohol without any water. Alcohol as manufactured by Indian distilleries is rectified spirit, which is 94.68% alcohol, and rest is water. It is not possible to remove remaining water from rectified spirit by straight distillation as ethyl alcohol forms a constant boiling mixture with water at this concentration and is known as azeotrope. Therefore, special process for removal of water is required for manufacture of absolute alcohol. In order to extract water from alcohol it is necessary to use some dehydrant or entrainer, which is capable of separating, water from alcohol. Simple dehydrant is unslacked lime, Industrial alcohol is taken in a rector and quick lime is added to that and the mixture is left over night for complete reaction. It is then distilled in fractionation column to get absolute alcohol. Water is retained by quick lime. This process is used for small-scale production of absolute alcohol by batch process.

Dehydration of alcohol/ethanol with entrainer process

For manufacture of absolute alcohol on large scale, Cyclohexane is used as entrainer. When 94.68% alcohol is mixed with Cyclohexane and distilled a ternary azeotrope is formed. The system consists of two to three columns. First is a dehydration column followed by recovery column. The Rectified spirit is fed into the dehydration column. Cyclohexane is also introduced in this column. Vapour of ethanol, water and cyclohexane close to its azeotropic concentration is collected from the top whereas absolute alcohol is collected from the bottom of the column. Ternary mixture of ethanol, water, and cyclohexane is condensed and sent for decantation where it forms two layers. Top one is cyclohexane rich layer whereas bottom layer is sent to recovery column. Water is collected from the bottom of the recovery column whereas ternary mixture of cyclohexane, water and ethanol comes out of the top, which is condensed and partially sent to dehydration column. Any cyclohexane lost in the system is taken care by adding make-up cyclohexane in the system. One thousand liters of industrial alcohol of 94% V/V contains 940 litres of absolute alcohol and 60 liters of water. For a capacity of 20 KLPD absolute alcohol plant make-ups cyclohexane required shall be 50 Kg. The cyclohexane is continuously recovered in the process and recycled as entrainer. About 20 to 30 liters of cyclohexane will be required every day to meet losses of cyclohexane in process. The process is rather simple and well established and given good quality of absolute alcohol.

In another method, glycerine is used as dehyrant. Glycerine is fed counter current wise to the rising alcohol vapours in a column. Glycerine absorbs all the water and leaves from the bottom of the column, which consist of Glycerine, water and some amount of alcohol. Distillate at the top is absolute alcohol glycerine water mixture is sent first to alcohol recovery column and then to vacuum evaporator for recovery of glycerine and removal of water. Glycerine is recycled. This process is also effective giving good quality of absolute alcohol.

Dehydration of alcohol/ethanol with molecular sieve process

The rectified spirit from the rectifier is superheated with steam in feed super heater. Superheated rectified spirit from feed super heater is passed to one of the pair of molecular sieve beds for several minutes. On a timed basis, the flow of superheated rectified spirit vapour is switched to the alternate bed of the pair. A moderate vacuum is applied by vacuum pump operating after condensation of the regenerated ethyl water mixture. This condensate is transferred from recycle drum to the Rectified Column in the hydrous distillation plant Via Recycle pump. The net make of anhydrous absolute alcohol draw is condensed in product condenser and passed to product storage. The detail flow sheet of alcohol/ethanol dehydration with molecular sieve distillation process is given in Figure 3.

Comparative statement of entrainer and molecular sieve process of dehydration of alcohol/ethanol.

Distillation based system	*Molecular sieve Dehydration*
Lower investment	Higher investment
Higher steam consumption	60% saving in steam consumption Higher power consumption
Degree of automation can vary as desired	Total automatic operation
Long life as distillation is sturdy process	Limited life primarily due to limited life of molecular sieve
Steady and uniform performance	The performance may vary over the period due to deterioration in the molecular sieve.
Solvent cyclohexane needs to be used as entrainer	No solvent is required
It is possible to remover part of the low boiling impurities from the feed	Almost all impurities in the feed would came along with absolute alcohol
Flexible in operation (operating capacity & purity wise)	Not so flexible. Design changes if absolute alcohol purity needs to be increased from 99.50% w/w to 99.90% w/w.
Less moving part, Low spares inventory	Need sophisticated components (PLC, automatic valves etc.) Required higher spare inventory.

Dehydration of alcohol/ethanol with Membrane Process

The development of system of dehydration with membrane for bulk removal has advantage of low operation cost. In this system, the arrangement of the dehydration and recovery column is the same with the cyclohexane dehydration. The rectified spirit is fed as liquid to a membrane unit. Where water and some alcohol vapour permeates through membrane. The driving force is pressure difference over the membrane. The permeate containing some alcohol flows back to the rectification column. As membrane is expensive, it is advantageous before dehydration to rectify alcohol to strength as high as possible to reduce the membrane cost.

The advantages of this system:

1. Easy operation,

2. Very low energy requirement per liter of absolute alcohol.

3. No toxic or hazardous chemical required.

However, this technology is not yet successfully proved on commercial scale in our country. In this industry, effluent produced is only water. Therefore, problems of pollution hazards are nil. Constant from Environmental Department and Pollution Control Board can be easily obtained as a matter of routine.

BIO-ETHANOL

Ethanol produced from biomass by using microorganisms such as *Saccharomyces cerevisiae* is known as bio ethanol. The beginning of bio ethanol use as petrol replacement was began in Brazil and USA during 1980s. At present, bio ethanol is not cost competitive as compared to petrol, but is being used for transport due to government subsidies. Any bio fuel proposed to be used for transport purpose should have following features:

1. It should be portable in sufficient quantities in the vehicle.
2. It should be burn in the internal combustion engines.
3. It should be roughly equivalent to petrol in energy content.

Desirable Characters of Bioethanol over Petrol

1. Bio ethanol has much higher latent heat of vaporization (855 MJ/Kg) than petrol (293 KJ/Kg). This energy is obtained from the air in the carburetor. As a result, the fuel mixture entering the cylinder is much cooler and hence denser in case of ethanol than in the case of petrol. Even though ethanol has only 61.8% (27.2 KJ/Kg) energy content of petrol (44 KJ/Kg), the energy produced by combustion of ethanol during each stroke is only slightly lower than that released from petrol.

2. Ethanol has a higher octane number (99) than petrol (80-100). As a result, "pre-ignition" does not occur when ethanol is used in engines set for petrol. Pre-ignition denotes ignition before the piston has reached the correct position during compression cycle. Pre-ignition leads to power loss and damage to valves and piston.

3. Ethanol is burnt more completely so that hydrocarbon omission is drastically lower as compared to that in case of petrol.

4. Higher octane rating of ethanol allows the compression ratio of the engines to be increased; results in increased production of power. In view of the above points, ethanol burning engines have only 10% more fuel consumption than petrol ones although ethanol has only about 62% as much energy content as petrol.

5. Ethanol has a much higher flash point (45°C) than petrol (13°C). Flashpoint is the temperature at which a substance catches fire. Therefore, ethanol is much less likely to catch fire and explode in cases of fuel leakage (e.g., during accidents).

6. It can be mixed with petrol; this increases the octane rating of petrol. In USA a 20% ethanol and 80% petrol mixture is being marketed as 'gasohol'. However, in such cases the ethanol must be 100% pure otherwise it will not mix in petrol and separation would occur.

7. Alcohol/ethanol is solar energy in liquid form. It can be made in large quantities from renewable sources.

8. The alcohol/ethanol production from agricultural material uses non-protein biomass. All protein can be extracted for human or livestock consumption/usages.

9. Road traffic is the major sources of pollution and produces substantial percentage of Non hydrocarbons, Co. Today all new are equipped with catalytic converter which are vary efficient in reducing the above pollutants by 90% in ideal conditions.

10. The burning of ethanol/alcohol forms no soot or carbon : carbon build up in an engine is eliminated.

There are some undesirable characters of bio-ethanol as compared to petrol.

1. Engines run on bio ethanol may give starting problems when the air is cool; this is because of the higher latent heat of evaporation of ethanol. This can be overcome by electrically heating the carburetor.

2. Bio ethanol is highly hydrophilic. As a result, it can absorb moisture from atmosphere etc. presence of water interferes with combustion and also causes corrosion in storage tanks and engines.

3. Bio ethanol reacts with metals used in the alloys of carburetor etc., e.g., aluminium and magnesium. It can be remedied by using nickel in the engine alloys.

4. The down stream processing for bio ethanol recovery is costly, as it requires lots of energy. This is perhaps the chief reason for limiting the use of bio ethanol as a fuel.

5. Bio ethanol run engines use about 10% more fuel than petrol, which means a proportionately larger tank.

6. Unlike petroleum product, ethanol/alcohol has no lubricating property hence additional lubricant like castor oil is required to mix with ethanol/alcohol for proper engine lubrication.

7. When ethanol burns in less quantity of air acetic acid is formed which causes corrosion in engines.

8. Combustion of ethanol/alcohol is likely to be complete due to when range of fuel air ratios, which results in an explosion. With alcohol/ethanol air fuel mixture found in partly empty storage tanks will probably be explosive. So special cellular fuel tank will have to be built for safety.

Technical Constraints and Corrective Action Points

A fleet aimed at studying the fuel economy and IIP and IOC (R&D) conducted drivability in case of ethanol-blended fuel and the results of these studies were shown below as blends:

1. Under city driving economy loss was 1% with 10% ethanol blended fuel and 3.90 percent with 20% ethanol blended fuel.

2. Low octane number and high self-ignition temperature makes ethanol/ alcohol unsuitable for diesel engines unless the fuel or the engine is modified to match the other.

3. Ethanol/alcohol and diesel are not miscible with each other and thus cannot be used as blend.

4. In gasoline 100% anhydrous alcohol would be preferred in the long run, which would make the use of blended fuel more uneconomical. A distillery producing ethanol under 1.5 percent water content costs about three times as much as a distillery to produce alcohol of 10% water by volume.

5. A long term continued availability of alcohols will be required to overcome any meaningful alco-fuel-programme and it has to be fully commercialized to get economical advantage that will require large commercial scale experimentation with alco-fuel, which has not so far been conducted.

6. In the Indian context no experimentation whatsoever has yet been conducted for finding our operational compatibility of motor engines to ethanol/alcohol/net alcohol as an oxygenator.

7. The production rate of ethanol/alcohol per ton of molasses or other sources is quite low (200 to 24 liters per tonne). Efforts should be directed to improve these yields to about 300 to 350 liters. Steps should be taken to produce alcohol from sources other than molasses, such as food grains, sweet sorghum, wood and waste cellulosic materials. Crops with high carbohydrates such as potatoes, corn etc. have theoretical alcohol/ethanol equivalent yield in excess of 2000 liters/hectare.

Sugarcane is indeed one of the most efficient biological converters of solar energy. Its photosynthetic efficiency is 3.8% as compared to earth's average (all vegetation inclusive) of 0.16% only. It has been estimated that 5.6 tonne of molasses (approximately 50% sugar) can yield 1 tonne of ethanol. Indian being the largest sugarcane country is in a better position with an area of 8.0 million hectares under sugarcane plantation and an average yield of 82.0 tons/hectares at 1990 level besides all agricultural crops and forests can be used to make ethanol / alcohol. Efficient conversion methodologies have to be developed to convert the huge renewable biomass resources base into usable value added products and alternative fuels or conventional fuel blending components for reformulated fuels. There is an essential need to formulate the integrated research and development programmes to produce ethanol / alcohol from cellulosic biomass and use the same efficiently for various applications.

Comparison of fuel properties of ethanol / alcohols and gasoline

Property	Methanol	Ethanol	Iso-Propanol/ Alcohol	Tert-Butyl Alcohol	Gasoline
Chemical formula	CH_3OH	C_2H_5OH	$(CH_3)_2CHOH$	$(CH_3)_3OH$	C_4 to C_{12}
Molecular weight	32.04	46.07	60.09	74.12	100 – 105
Composition, wt. %					
Carbon	37.5	52.2	60.0	64.8	85.88
Hydrogen	12.6	13.1	13.4	13.6	12.15
Oxygen	49.9	34.7	26.6	21.6	0.0
Sp.gr. 60°F /60°F	0.796	0.794	0.789	0.791	0.72 – 0.78
Density, lb/gal @ 60°F	6.63	6.61	6.57	6.59	6.0 – 6.5
Boiling temp. °F	149	172	180	181	80.437
Reid vapour pressure, psi	4.6	2.3	1.8	1.8	8.15
Water solubility, @ 60°F					
Fuel in water, volume %	100	100	100	100	Negligible
Water in fuel, volume %	100	100	100	100	Negligible
Viscosity, centipoises @ 68°F	0.59	1.19	2.38	4.2	0.37 – 0.44
Flash point, closed cup. °F	52	55	53	52	45
Auto ignition, temp. °F	867	793	750	892	495
Flammability limits, volume %					
Lower	7.3	4.3	2.0	2.4	1.4
Higher	36.0	19.0	12.0	8.0	7.6
Latent heat of vaporization, Btu/gal @ 60°F	3340	2378	2100	1700	-900
Heating value, lower (liquid-fuel-water vapour) Btu/gal @ 60°F	56800	76000	87400	94100	109000
Stoichiometric air-fuel weight	6.45	9.00	10.3	11.1	14.7
Ratio moles product/ moles $O_2 + N_2$	1.21	1.12	1.10	1.10	1.08

Features of various biofuels, which can be produced by using biotechnology on large scale.

Biofuel	Substrate	Microorganism(s)	Status of production	Limiting factors
Ethanol	Starch, sugar crops	Bacillus licheniformisS cerevisie. Zymomonas	Billions of litres/yr	Low productivity (Brazil)High substrate cost (USA)
	Cellulose wastesa. Enzyme hydrolysis	Trichoderma reeseiS. CerevisieRecombinant E. coliClostridium sp. Fusarium oxysporum	Likely to enter commercial scale production; suited for energy crops	Low yieldsSlow rate of productionPretreatment needed
	b. Acid hydrolysis	S cerevisie. Zymomonas	Likely to enter commercial production; comparable to enzymatic process; suited for waste materials	Low yieldsHigh acid recycling costs
	c. From synthesis gas	Clostridium liungdahlii	Preliminary stages of development	Mass transfer limitations in bioreactor
Methane	Farm and human wastes; municipal solid wastes; effluents from food and dairy industries etc.	A group of anaerobic microorganisms	Widely used	Slow ratesEconomically unattractive as transport fuel
Butanol	Soluble carbohydrates	Clostridium acetobutylicum, C. beijernickii	Commercial production possible in near future for use as an additive in gasoline	Low product toleranceHigh product cost
Hydrogen	Sunlight and water	Chlamydomonas reinhardtii C. moewusii	Long-term research and development needed	Efficiency declines with high light intensities
	Sugars and fatty acids (starch & cellulose)	Anaerobic bacteria like Clostridium	-	-
Biodiesel	Sunlight and CO_2	Monraphidium minutum, Cyclotella crypticum Euphorbian plants,Copaifera tree etc.	Long-term research and development needed	Lack of a genetic transformation system

BIO-ETHANOL PRODUCTION

At present, there are three important routes for producing bio ethanol:

1. From starch or sugar crops,
2. From cellulose following enzymatic hydrolysis, and
3. From cellulose following chemical hydrolysis.

The cost of production of bioethanol from the three routes is comparable. However, commercial production is based on starch and sugar crops only; there is no full-scale production plant based on cellulose.

Billions of liters of bio ethanol is produced annually mostly in Brazil (from sugarcane) and USA (from maize). The process based on sugarcane has low productivity and the enormous amount of cellulosic bagasse is either burnt or ploughed back into soil; this biomass is a potential source of bio ethanol.

Sugarcane, Sugar beet, Sweet sorghum etc. provide a good substrate. Juices from these crops contain sugar, e.g., sugarcane juice has about 12% fermentable sugars, and can be used directly for fermentation. Molasses, sweet sorghum syrup and spent sulphite liquor are the most common substrates. Molasses (C grade) obtained after sugar recovery contains about 35% sucrose, 19% other reducing agents and 14% other organic substances; thus the total fermentable sugars are nearly 50-55%. Molasses is first suitably diluted, then treated with 0.5% by weight concentrated sulphuric acid at 70-95°C (mainly for removal of calcium salts and acidification) and used for fermentation. Cereals like maize, wheat, sorghum etc. contain 60-75% w/w starch, which on hydrolysis produces glucose in the ratio 9:10 (Figure 4).

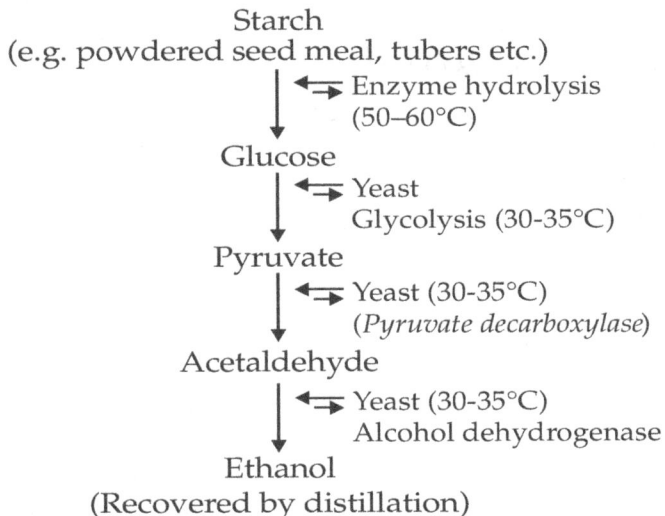

Starch
(e.g. powdered seed meal, tubers etc.)
↓ ⇌ Enzyme hydrolysis
(50–60°C)
Glucose
↓ ⇌ Yeast
Glycolysis (30-35°C)
Pyruvate
↓ ⇌ Yeast (30-35°C)
(*Pyruvate decarboxylase*)
Acetaldehyde
↓ ⇌ Yeast (30-35°C)
Alcohol dehydrogenase
Ethanol
(Recovered by distillation)

Flow chart for the production of ethanol from a starch substrate.

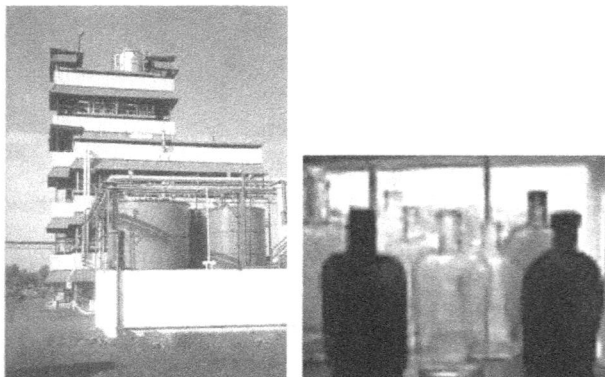

Generally, starch is a mixture of amylose (20-30%; water soluble linear polymer) and amylopectin (70-80%; water insoluble branched polymer). A cooking process aided by enzymes usually achieves conversion of starch into glucose. Seeds are powdered and the resulting meal is mixed with water in the ratio of 1:2.5 - 3. α-amylase is then added and the temperature is raised by steam injection to 105-110°C and held for about 20 min. During this period, starch grains become dissolved to form a viscous suspension (gelatinization) due to the cooking effect of heat. At the same time α-amylase digests partially some of the starch molecules; this reduces the viscosity of the suspension; this is called liquefaction. The suspension contains solubilized starch molecules, and dextrins (short chains of glucose units). The suspension called mash is cooled to 85-90°C and more α-amylase is added to complete the process of liquification (for 90 min). The total dose of α-amylase is about 1.5 kg/tonne starch. The mash is cooled to 55-60°C and 1.5-3.5 liter glucoamylase/tonne of starch is added to produce glucose from dextrins and maltose. The reaction duration is usually 2 days, and it achieves the dextrose equivalent of 99. Saccharification by glucoamylase continues during the fermentation.

Proper fermentation of 100 g glucose by selected strains of *Saccharomyces cerevisiae* and *Saccharomyces carlsbergensis* yields 45-49 g bio ethanol, the theoretical limit being 51.1 g.

($C_6H_{12}O_6$ $2C_2H_5OH$ + $2CO_2$). For the fermentation process batch or continuous processes are used. Batch process is the most commonly used. Ammonium sulphate or Urea (N source) and a salt of phosphoric acid (P source) are added to the substrate. Most commonly the temperature during fermentation is 32-38°C and pH is between 4.5-5.0.

As the ethanol level rises, both ethanol production and yeast cell growth are progressively inhibited, and eventually cells begin to die.

In general, yeast growth stops at 6-9% w/v ethanol, but ethanol production, at least in some strains, may continue upto 15% ethanol or higher. Ethanol inhibition can be relieved by continuous removal of ethanol. Ethanol recovery is based on distillation.

(a) The broth is distilled in a beer column to yield 85% v/v ethanol.

(b) The next step of rectification gives 96.5% ethanol, which is then.

(c) Dehydrated to 99.4% using benzene or cyclohexane if the ethanol is to be used as a fuel blend.

The wastewater effluent can be used directly on land, used for anaerobic digestion for methane generation, evaporated to dry syrup for animal feed or fuel or used as substrate for fungal biomass production.

Future look out for bio-ethanol production

1. To increase the substrate utilization ability of excellent ethanol produces like yeast and *Zymomonas mobilis.*

2. To enhance alcohol tolerance of yeast.

3. To increase the bio ethanol production ability of bacteria capable of utilizing cellulose, hemicellulose, pentoses etc.

4. Practical exploitation of the superior capabilities of *zymomonas mobilis.*

5. Efficient and cost effective process of continuous recovery of ethanol needs to be developed.

6. More efficient and cheaper methods of ethanol recovery need to be developed to reduce the cost of recovery. Some possible approaches may be reverse osmosis, selective adsorption using solid adsorbents and use of supercritical CO_2 to selectively extract ethanol.

Biotechnology in bio-ethanol production

The potential areas where biotechnology can make a notable contribution are:

(a) Development of more efficient organisms for alcoholic fermentation,

(b) Devising a more efficient use of these microorganisms, e.g., in cell immobilized systems,

(c) To develop organisms capable of utilizing cellulose and hemicellulose present in corn and other sugar crops, and

(d) Practical exploitation of the advantageous features of *zymomonas mobilis.*

Recovery of bio-ethanol from biomass

Recovery of ethanol from the fermentation broth is by distillation, which exploits the difference in boiling points of ethanol (87°C) and water (100°C). As a result, when a water ethanol mixture having 95% ethanol is heated, the vapour has a greater concentration of ethanol than the liquid phase. Thus a dilute ethanol : water mixture can be repeatedly distilled to obtain more concentrated (upto 95%) ethanol solution. The principle of sequential distillation is used in a cylindrical distillation column, which is divided into a series of chambers by perforated plates. The ethanol water mixture is boiled using steam and the vapour rises into the column. Essentially, each chamber of the column functions as a distillation unit so that the proportion of alcohol goes on sequentially increasing as it rises to the upper chambers of the column. A properly designed column would yield 95% ethanol from its top most chambers. Such a column can be run either in a batch or in continuous mode.

When 95% ethanol is heated, the proportion of water present in the vapour phase is the same as that in the liquid phase. Therefore, simple distillation is no more helpful in further purification/concentration of ethanol. A small amount of benzene is added to 95% ethanol, which is then distilled. The distillate is nearly 100% ethanol, and the benzene can also be recovered. Thus recovery of pure ethanol requires considerable amounts of energy, which raises its production cost; this has been the chief reason for the limited use of this valuable biofuel/ bio ethanol for transport purposes.

Concluding remarks

Wiser use of energy, land and raw materials is a prerequisite for stable; sustainable and economic agriculture sustainable food and nutrition security involves meeting current needs in agricultural production without sacrificing the prospects for meeting the needs of future generations. Wiser use of biotechnology can be a great help to achieve this goal.

REFERENCES

Baldwin, T.O., Raushel, F.M. and Scott, A.I. 1991. *Chemical Aspects of Enzyme Biotechnology-Fundamentals.* (eds.) Plenum Press, New York.

Balkwill, F.R. 1989. *Cytokines in Cancer Therapy.* Oxford University Press, Oxford.

Bernarde, M.A. 1992. Global Warming – Global Warming. John Wiley and Sons, Chichester.

Bhojwani, S.S. (ed.) 1990. *Plant Tissue Culture: Applications and Limitations.* Elsevier, Amsterdam.

Bhojwani, S.S. and Razdan, M.K. 1983. *Plant Tissue Culture: Theory and Practice.* Elsevier, Amsterdam.

Bose, Bandana. 2005. *Developments in Physiology, Biochemistry and Molecular Biology of Plants* Vol. 1. New India Publishing Agency (NIPA) New Delhi.

Bose, Bandana. 2008. *Developments in Physiology, Biochemistry and Molecular Biology of Plants* Vol. 2. New India Publishing Agency (NIPA) New Delhi.

Brinster, R.L. 1993. *Stem cells and transgenic mice in the study of development.* Int. J. Dev. Bio. 37: 89-99.

Bu'lock, J.D. and Kristiansen, B. 1987. *Basic Biotechnology.* Academic Press, London.

Campbell, R.W. and Howell, J.A. 1995. *Comprehensive Biotechnology.* Pergamon Press, Oxford.

Chandra, S. 2006. *Biotechnology of VA Mycorrhizza: Indian Scenario.* New India Publishing Agency (NIPA) New Delhi.

Chaplin, M.F. and Bucke, C. 1990. *Enzyme Technology.* Cambridge University Press, Cambridge.

Darwin, Henry. 2009. *Illustrated Plant Pathology: Basic Concepts.* New India Publishing Agency (NIPA) New Delhi.

Darwin, Henry. 2011. *Crop Diseases: Identification, Treatment and Management.* New India Publishing Agency (NIPA) New Delhi.

Demain, A.L. and Solomon, N.A. (eds.) 1986. *Industrial Microbiology and Biotechnology.* American Society for Microbiology, Washington, DC.

Dietrich Knorr (ed.) 1987. *Food Biotechnology.* Marcel Dekker, INC, New York.

Dutta and Dutta. 2011. *Experimental Biotechnology: Practical Manual Series* Vol. 6. New India Publishing Agency (NIPA) New Delhi.

Fletcher, G.L. and Davies, P.L. 1991. *Transgenic fish for acquaculture.* In J. K. Setlow (ed.) Genetic Engineering, Vol. 13, pp. 331-370. Plenum Press, New York.

Garrow, J.S. and James, J.S. 1998. *Human Nutrition and Dietetics.* Churchill Living Stone, Edinburgh, UK.

Gatehouse, A.M.R., Hilder, V.A. and Boulter, D. (eds.) 1992. *Plant Genetic Manipulation for Crop Protection.* CAB International, Walling ford, UK.

Gibbs, D.F. and Bucke, C. 1983. *Biotechnology, Chemical Feedstock and Energy Utilization.* Frances Printer (Publ.), Washington, DC.

Gibbs, D.F. and Greenhalgh, M.E. 1983. *Biotechnology, Chemical Feedstocks and Energy Utilization.* Francis Pinter (Publ.), London.

Gregoriadis, G. 1989. Targeting of Drugs: *Implications in Medicine.* Wiley, New York.

Grierson, D. 1991. *Plant Genetic Engineering, Plant Biotechnology* Vol. 1, Blackie, Glasgow.

Goding, J.W. 1993. *Monoclonal Antibodies: Principles and Practice* (3rd edn.) Academic Press, New York.

Gupta, P.K. 2000. *Elements of Biotechnology.* Rastogi Publications, Meerut, India.

Gupta, M.L. and Jangir, M.L. 2002. *Cell Biology: Fundamentals and Applications.* Agribios, Jodhapur, India.

Hazra, Pranab. 2011. *Modern Technology in Vegetable Production.* New India Publishing Agency (NIPA) New Delhi.

Hobson, P.N. and Whately, A.D. 1993. *Anaerobic Digestion, Modern Theory and Practice.* Elsevier, London.

Jain, S.M., Sopory, S.K. and Veilleux, R.E. 1996. *In vitro Haploid Production in Higher Plants.* Vol. 1. *Fundamental Aspects,* Vol. 2. *Applications,* Vol. 3. *Important Selected Plants,* Vol. 4. *Cereals,* Vol. 5. *Oil, Ornamental and Miscellaneous Plants.* Kluwer Academic Publishers, London.

Jain, Vanitha. 2011. *Nitrogen Use Efficiency in Plants.* New India Publishing Agency (NIPA) New Delhi.

Kader, A.A. (ed.) 1992. *Post-harvest Technology of Horticultural Crops.* 2nd edn. University of California, Davis, USA.

Keshvachandran. 2007. *Recent Trends in Horticultural Biotechnology:* In 2 Vols. New India Publishing Agency (NIPA) New Delhi.

Kirby, L.T. 1990. *Fingerprinting: An Introduction,* Stockton, New York.

Kumar, N. 2006. *Breeding of Horticultural Crops: Principles and Practices.* New India Publishing Agency (NIPA) New Delhi.

Kurian, A. 2007. *Commercial Crops Technology:* Vol. 08. *Horticulture Science Series.* New India Publishing Agency (NIPA) New Delhi.

Kurian, A. 2007. *Medicinal Plants*: Vol. 2. *Horticulture Science Series.* New India Publishing Agency (NIPA) New Delhi.

Lal, R. and Lal, S. 1990. *Crop Improvement Utilizing Biotechnology.* CRC Press, Boca Raton, Florida, USA.

Leach, C.K. and Van Dam-Mieras, M, C.E. (eds.) 1994. *Biotechnological Innovations in Energy and Environmental Management.* Butterworth-Heinemann Ltd., Oxford.

Leach, C.K. and Van Dam-Mieras, M, C.E. (eds.) 1994. *Biotechnological Innovations in Environmental Management.* Butterworth-Heinemann Ltd., Oxford (BIOTOL series).

Lewin, B. 1994. Genes V. Oxford University Press, New York.

Lynd, L.R., Cushman, J.H., Nichols, R.J. and Wyman, C.E. 1991. *Fuel ethanol from cellulosic biomass.* Science. 251: 1381-1323.

Meyers, R.A. 1995. *Molecular Biology and Biotechnology: A Comprehensive Desk Reference.* VCH Publishier (UK) Ltd., Cambridge.

Moss, J.P. 1992. *Biotechnology for Crop Improvement in Asia*. ICRISAT, Patancheru, India.

Narayanasamy, P. 2011. *Crop Diseases Management: Principles and Practices*. New India Publishing Agency (NIPA) New Delhi.

Old, R.W. and Primrose, S.B. 1990. *Principles of Gene manipulation, An Introduction to Genetic Engineering*. Blackwell Sci. Publ., London

Parakhia, M.V. 2010. *Molecular Biology and Biotechnology: Microbial Method*. New India Publishing Agency (NIPA) New Delhi.

Pare, Aakas. 2011. *Food Process Engineering and Technology*. New India Publishing Agency (NIPA) New Delhi.

Patel, Sunil. 2010. *Handbook of Life Sciences*. New India Publishing Agency (NIPA) New Delhi.

Peter, C.M. and Bryce, J.H. (eds.) 2004. *Cereal Biotechnology*. CRC, Boca Raton, Boston New York, Washington, DC.

Peter, K.V.: eds. 2011. *The Science of Horticulture* Vol. 1. New India Publishing Agency (NIPA) New Delhi.

Peter, K.V.: eds. 2011. *The Science of Horticulture* Vol. 2. New India Publishing Agency (NIPA) New Delhi.

Pinkert, C.A. 1994. *Transgenic Animal Technology: A Laboratory Handbook*. Academic Press, San Diego, CA.

Purdon, P.W. 1990. *Environment Health*. Academic Press, London.

Ram, Hari Har. 2007. *Genetic Resources and Seed Enterprises: Management and Policies: In 2 Parts*. New India Publishing Agency (NIPA) New Delhi.

Rana, Mahesh. 2011. *Breeding and Protection of Vegetables*. New India Publishing Agency (NIPA) New Delhi.

Rana, Mahesh. 2011. *Physio-Biochemistry and Biotechnology of Vegetable Crops*. New India Publishing Agency (NIPA) New Delhi.

Rai, Nagendra. 2006. *Heterosis Breeding in Vegetable Crops*. New India Publishing Agency (NIPA) New Delhi.

Roy, Bidhan. 2009. *Abiotic Stress Tolerance in Crop Plants: Breeding and Biotechnology*. New India Publishing Agency (NIPA) New Delhi.

Roy, A.K. 2010. *Laboratory Manual of Microbiology: Practical Manual Series* : 05. New India Publishing Agency (NIPA) New Delhi.

Sabina, George. 2010. *Ornamental Plants*. New India Publishing Agency (NIPA) New Delhi.

Saikai, Ratul. 2008. *Microbial Biotechnology*. New India Publishing Agency (NIPA) New Delhi.

Salunkhe, D.K., Chavan, J.K., Adsule, R.N. and Kadam, S.S. (eds.) 1992. *World Oilseeds: Chemistry, Technology and Utilization*. VNR, New Delhi.

Salunkhe, D.K., Chavan, J.K. and Kadam, S.S. (eds.) 1985. *Post-harvest Biotechnology of Legumes*. CRC Press, Florida, USA.

Salunkhe, D.K. and Kadam, S.S. 2000. *Handbook of Fruits and Vegetables. Marcel Dekker*, New York.

Salunkhe, D.K., Kadam, S.S. and Chavan, J.K. (eds.) 1985. *Post-harvest Biotechnology of Cereals*. CRC Press, Florida, USA.

Sharma, S.K. 2010. *Postharvest Management and Processing of Fruits and Vegetables:* Instant Notes. New India Publishing Agency (NIPA) New Delhi.

Sharma, Girish. 2009. *Systematics of Fruit Crops.* New India Publishing Agency (NIPA) New Delhi.

Sheela, V.L. 2008. *Flowers for Trade:* Vol. 10. *Horticulture Science Series.* New India Publishing Agency (NIPA) New Delhi.

Shukla, Y.M. 2009. *Plant Secondary Metabolites.* New India Publishing Agency (NIPA) New Delhi.

Singer, M. and Berg, P. 1991. *Genes and Genomes.* University Science Books, Mill Valley, California and Blackwell Sci. Publ., Oxford.

Singh, A.K. 2006. *Flower Crops: Cultivation and Management.* New India Publishing Agency (NIPA) New Delhi.

Singh, B.D. 2000. *Biotechnology.* Kalayani Publisher, Ludhiana.

Smith, R.H. and Hood, E.E. 1995. *Agrobacterium tumefaciens transformation of monocotyledons.* Crop Sci. 35: 301-309.

Srivastava. 2010. *Modern Methods in Plant Physiology.* New India Publishing Agency (NIPA) New Delhi.

Swamy, V.M.K. 1995. *Opportunities in biotechnology and instrumentation.* Biotech. Dev. Rev. June-Dec. 1995: 48-52.

Thacker, J.R.M. 1993/94. *Transgenic Crop Plants and Pest Control Sci. Progress.* 77: 207-219.

Thara, K.M. 2009. *Biotechnology: Practical Manual Series,* Vol. 4. New India Publishing Agency (NIPA) New Delhi.

Timir B.J. and Biswajit, G. 2005. *Plant Tissue Culture: Basic and Applied.* Universities Press.

Tomar, R.S. 2009. *Molecular Markers and Plant Biotechnology.* New India Publishing Agency (NIPA) New Delhi.

Tomar and Patel. 2009. *Handbook of Genetics and Biotechnology.* New India Publishing Agency (NIPA) New Delhi.

Trends in Biotechnology Vol. 13, Sep., 1995, pp. 313-409.

Veisser, R. G. F. and Jacobsen, E. 1993. *Towards modifying Plants for altered starch content and composition.* TIBTECH 11: 63-68.

Verma, V.R. and Joshi, V.K. 2000. *Post-harvest Technology of Fruits and Vegetables.* Vol. II. Indus, New Delhi.

Vasil, I.K. and Thorpe, T.A. (eds.) 1994. *Plant Cell and Tissue Culture.* Kluwer Academic Publishers, London.

Waugh, R. and Powell, W. 1992. *Using RAPD markers for crop improvement.* TIBTECH 10: 186-191.

Zaitlin, M., Day, P. and Hollaender, A. (eds.) 1985. *Biotechnology in Plant Science, Relevance to Agriculture in the Eighties.* Academic Press, New York.

www.ingramcontent.com/pod-product-compliance
Lightning Source LLC
Chambersburg FA
CBHW021435180326

41458CB00001B/289